Pocket Guide
of ICD-10-CM
and
ICD-10-PCS

Ann M. Zeisset, RHIT, CCS, CCS-P,
and Sue Bowman, RHIA, CCS

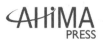

ISBN 978-1-58426-252-7
AHIMA Product No. AC203010

Claire Blondeau, MBA, SENIOR EDITOR
Ashley Sullivan, ASSISTANT EDITOR
Katie Greenock, EDITORIAL/PRODUCTION
COORDINATOR
Ken Zielske, DIRECTOR OF PUBLICATIONS

American Health Information Management Association
233 North Michigan Avenue, 21st Floor
Chicago, Illinois 60601-5800
www.ahima.org

Contents

CONTENTS

About the Authors

Ann M. Zeisset, RHIT, CCS, CCS-P, is the Manager of Professional Practice Resources for the American Health Information Management Association (AHIMA). Zeisset provides professional expertise on coding practice issue to AHIMA members, the media, and outside organizations. She also authors and supports AHIMA online coding education (including the "Coding Basics" program), is a technical advisor for the Association on ICD-9-CM and CPT coding publications, and is the author of several publications.

Zeisset authored *Advanced CPT/HCPCS for Physician Office Coding and Applying Inpatient Coding Skills under Prospective Payment*, published by AHIMA, and is a contributing author for *Healthcare Code Sets, Clinical Terminologies, and Classification Systems* and the *Clinical Coding Workout: Practice Exercises for Skill Development* coding reference textbooks.

Prior to joining AHIMA in 1999, Zeisset served in various director and coding roles. She has been an educator of coding and HIM for more than 20 years at multiple colleges. Zeisset has authored many coding-related articles and has presented numerous seminars and educational sessions on coding and other HIM related topics throughout the United States including many for Home Health professionals. Zeisset was also awarded the Distinguished Member award from SILHIMA in 2003 and the

Certified Coding Specialist award in 2005.

Zeisset recently completed a one year contract between the Foundation for Research and Education and CMS to determine potential impacts to CMS when converting from ICD-9-CM to ICD-10-CM/PCS coding systems. Zeisset is a frequent author and speaker on ICD-10-CM/PCS and serves as faculty for AHIMA's Academy for ICD-10. Zeisset received a bachelor's degree in Organizational Leadership at Greenville College.

Sue Bowman, RHIA, CCS, is director of Coding Policy and Compliance for AHIMA, a position she has held since 1995. She leads all AHIMA policy initiatives related to coding practice and fraud and abuse prevention and serves as AHIMA's representative to the Cooperating Parties, a group with direct input on the creation, maintenance, and updating of healthcare codes and guidelines.

Bowman is a leader in AHIMA's advocacy initiatives for the U.S. adoption and use of standard classifications and terminologies, including ICD-10-CM/PCS and SNOMED-CT. She authored AHIMA's white paper on the coordination of SNOMED-CT and ICD-10 in an electronic health record environment. Bowman is also the editor of an AHIMA publication titled "Health Information Management Compliance: Guidelines for Preventing Fraud and Abuse." She participates in a variety of AHIMA activities pertaining to the advancement of healthcare data quality and the use of healthcare data standards.

Bowman has provided input on the development of the ICD-10-CM/PCS coding systems and associated resources, including the *ICD-10-CM Official Guidelines for Coding and Reporting*, CMS' ICD-10 fact sheets, and the General Equivalence Mapping users' guides. She coauthored AHIMA's ICD-10 Preparation Checklist and has served as a speaker for CMS' ICD-10 outreach calls. Bowman has written many articles and given a number of presentations on the topic of ICD-10. She also serves on the World Health Organization's morbidity reference group, which develops international rules and guidelines for the use of ICD-10 and ICD-11.

Prior to taking her position with AHIMA in 1995, Bowman served as director of Utilization Review and Data Quality at St. Mary's Hospital in Centralia, Illinois. She also has served as a member of the Board of Directors of the Illinois Health Information Management Association and as past chair of AHIMA's Society for Clinical Coding.

Bowman received a Bachelor of Science degree in Medical Record Administration from Daemen College in Amherst, NY.

Preface

This book is a quick reference guide to key information about ICD-10-CM/PCS for anyone involved in ICD-10-CM/PCS transition planning and preparation, including health information management and coding professionals, information technology personnel, vendors, healthcare data analysts, and other data users.

The scope and complexity of the transition to ICD-10-CM/PCS are significant. This transition to ICD-10-CM/PCS will be a transformational effort affecting many systems, processes, and people. It will have a tremendous and pervasive impact on every operational process across a healthcare-related business. Ready access to key information about ICD-10-CM/PCS is an important aspect of effective and efficient transition preparation.

This book provides an overview of the structure, logic, organization, and unique features of ICD-10-CM/PCS and the similarities and differences between these code sets and ICD-9-CM, in a concise, easy-to-use format. Information on the development of the General Equivalence Maps (GEMs) and how to use them as a tool to accurately and effectively translate large amounts of data from ICD-9-CM to ICD-10-CM/PCS is also included. The book describes the limitations of maps and data trending challenges due to the significant differences between the old and new code sets. High-level guidance on the impact of the transition to ICD-10-CM/PCS and key preparatory activities is provided as well.

The content summarizes the information that would most likely be needed by individuals wishing to gain a basic familiarity with the new codes and those involved directly in ICD-10-CM/PCS transition activities. The book can be used to orient vendors and in-house information technology staff and others affected by the transition on the specifications of ICD-10-CM/PCS that they will need to know to implement systems changes, database conversions, report and form modifications, and other changes required by the transition to the new code sets. It can also be used as a reference by data users wishing to gain a general knowledge of the impact of the transition on data comparability and data trending challenges. When an answer to a basic question about ICD-10-CM/PCS, transition preparation, and mapping between the old and new code sets is needed quickly, the information is at one's fingertips in this Pocket Guide.

Chapter 1
Overview of ICD-10

International Classification of Diseases 9th Revision Clinical Modification

The ICD-9-CM code set is the U.S. clinical modification of the World Health Organization's (WHO) International Classification of Diseases 9th Revision (ICD-9) diagnosis classification system. ICD has become the international, standard diagnostic classification for all general epidemiological and many health management purposes. The purpose of ICD is to permit the systematic recording, analysis, interpretation, and comparison of mortality and morbidity data collected in different countries. The United States has clinically modified the ICD-9 WHO classification system (ICD-9-CM)

The Health Care Financing Administration (HCFA), now known as the Centers for Medicare & Medicaid Services (CMS), developed a procedure coding system to accompany the ICD-9-CM diagnosis coding system. The ICD-9-CM coding system was implemented in the United States in 1979. ICD-9-CM diagnosis codes are used by all healthcare providers, whereas ICD-9-CM procedure codes are only used for facility reporting of hospital inpatient services.

Although diagnostic and procedural coding for statistics and research was the original function of the system, since 1983, ICD-9-CM also has been used to communicate information on healthcare services for the purpose of reimbursement.

There are many uses of coded data, such as:

- Classifying morbidity and mortality information for statistical purposes
- Indexing hospital records by disease and operations
- Reporting diagnoses and procedures for reimbursement
- Storing and retrieving data
- Determining patterns of care among healthcare providers
- Analyzing payments for health services
- Performing epidemiological studies, clinical trials, and clinical research
- Measuring quality, safety, and efficacy of care
- Designing payment systems
- Setting health policy
- Monitoring resource utilization
- Implementing operational and strategic plans
- Designing healthcare delivery systems
- Improving clinical, financial, and administrative performance
- Preventing and detecting healthcare fraud and abuse
- Tracking public health and risks

HIPAA Code Sets

In 2000, the U.S. Department of Health and Human Services (HHS) published final regulations for electronic transactions and code set standards promulgated under the Health Insurance Portability and Accountability Act of 1996 (HIPAA). The ICD-9-CM diagnosis codes were adopted as the code set standard for reporting diseases, injuries, impairments, and other health problems and their manifestations, as well as causes of injury and disease impairment, in all healthcare settings. The ICD-9-CM procedure codes were adopted as the code set standard for reporting procedures or other actions taken for diseases, injuries, and impairments of hospital inpatients reported by hospitals and related to prevention, diagnosis, treatment, and management. Although the ICD-9-CM code sets were already in common use, the HIPAA regulations set standards for their use and also named the *ICD-9-CM Official Guidelines for Coding and Reporting* a component of the code set standard. This makes adherence to the ICD-9-CM guidelines a requirement for compliance with the rule.

Data Uses

The need for greater coding accuracy and specificity has increased considerably since the implementation of ICD-9-CM. ICD-9-CM is used for many more purposes today than when it was originally developed and is no longer able to support today's health information needs. Developed in the 1970s, the ICD-9-CM code set no longer fits with the twenty-first century healthcare system and can no longer fulfill the need for accurate and complete healthcare data in the United States. For example, when prospective payment systems came into existence, the concerns for data quality, coding education, and medical record documentation received new emphasis. The consequences of inaccurate claims data in a fee-for-service environment had not been nearly as critical. Many reimbursement systems that are not based on a prospective payment methodology also require complete, accurate, and detailed coding in order to negotiate or calculate appropriate reimbursement rates, determine coverage, and establish medical necessity.

ICD-9-CM Outdated

ICD-9-CM terminology and classifications are outdated and inconsistent with current medical practice. Also, the system is rapidly running out of space and cannot accommodate the addition of new codes to address advances in medical knowledge or technology, or newly identified diseases. In some cases, proposals for new codes have not been implemented simply because there is insufficient space for a new code. ICD-9-CM codes also lack sufficient clinical detail to describe the severity or complexity of diagnoses, and the system does not provide sufficient codes for healthcare encounters for reasons other than treatment of disease or injury, such as preventive medicine. Our ability to effectively perform the following healthcare activities has been seriously hindered by our failure to replace ICD-9-CM with a modern classification system:

- Measure quality of care
- Identify medical errors and patient safety issues
- Track public health threats, such as avian flu
- Evaluate resource utilization
- Exchange meaningful health data with other organizations and government agencies
- Initiate pay-for-performance

The need to replace ICD-9-CM in the United States was identified in the early 1990s, when the National Committee on Vital and Health Statistics (NCVHS) reported that ICD-9-CM was rapidly becoming outdated and recommended immediate United States commitment to developing a migration to ICD-10 for morbidity and mortality coding. CMS (then HCFA) recommended that steps should be taken to improve the flexibility of ICD-9-CM or replace it with a more flexible option sometime after the year 2000.

Development of ICD-10

The WHO owns and publishes the international version of the ICD classification system. The purpose of the ICD classification system is to promote international agreement on the collection, classification, processing, and presentation of health data, including both mortality and morbidity data, so that health data from around the world can be meaningfully compared. In everyday practice, ICD has become an international diagnostic classification system used for all general epidemiological and healthcare purposes. In 1992, the WHO published the tenth revision of the ICD system (ICD-10), which represents the broadest scope of any ICD revision to date. The goal of the tenth revision was to expand the content, purpose, and scope of the system. It was designed to include ambulatory care services, increase clinical detail, capture risk factors in primary care, identify emergent diseases, and develop group diagnoses for epidemiological purposes. ICD-10 provides many more categories for disease and other health-related conditions than previous revisions through its alphanumeric coding scheme. In addition, it includes chapter rearrangements, additions and revisions, and extensive changes to the mental and behavioral disorders, the injury, poisoning, and certain other consequences of external causes, and the external causes of morbidity and mortality. It also includes additional categories for postprocedural disorders.

Today, ICD-10 is used to record both mortality and morbidity data by many countries. The United States is the only industrialized country which has not implemented ICD-10 for morbidity reporting. The World Health Organization's ICD-10 has been used in the United States to report mortality data since 1999.

Having an international coding system provides a way in which data can be collected, analyzed, interpreted, and compared.

Development of ICD-10-CM and ICD-10-PCS

ICD-10-CM is the U.S. clinical modification of the WHO's ICD-10 classification system. Because the United States is required to report mortality and morbidity data to the WHO under an agreement that is similar to an international treaty, any revisions made to the tenth revision of the system must conform to ICD-10 conventions. As owner and publisher of ICD-10, the WHO promotes the development of any adaptations that will expand the usefulness and comparability of health statistics. Therefore, the WHO has authorized an adaptation of ICD-10 (ICD-10-CM) for use in the United States. Both the WHO version of ICD-10 and the U.S. ICD-10-CM contain diagnostic codes but no procedure codes.

ICD-10-CM

The U.S. clinical modification (ICD-10-CM) was developed by the National Center for Health Statistics (NCHS), a division of the Centers for Disease Control and Prevention (CDC). The NCHS has worked closely with many organizations to address the clinical needs in the United States to incorporate the level of detail needed in a morbidity classification and to provide code titles and language that complement accepted clinical practice for all users in the United States. ICD-10-CM has 68,069 codes, whereas there are 14,025 ICD-9-CM diagnosis codes.

ICD-10-PCS

ICD-10-PCS was developed in the United States under contract by CMS to replace the ICD-9-CM procedural coding system. It is not derived from an international coding system, but is designed to reflect the use of current and future technology changes. The objectives of ICD-10-PCS were to improve accuracy and efficiency of coding, reduce training efforts, and improve communication with physicians. The development of ICD-10-PCS had as its goal the incorporation of four essential attributes: completeness, expandability, standard-ized terminology, and a multi-axial structure. ICD-10-PCS has 72,589 codes, whereas there are 3,824 ICD-9-CM procedure codes.

Comments and Testing

The development of both ICD-10-CM and ICD-10-PCS has included significant input from stake-holder groups. After initial development, public comments on these code sets were solicited and they underwent testing. Testing has demonstrated the benefits of the new code sets and the fact that a greater number of codes does not necessarily increase the difficulty in learning to use the systems. The results of the testing of both code sets led to some modifications to the code sets themselves as well as the guidelines for their use. In the years since initial system development, there have been opportunities for the public to provide comments. The developers of both code sets have provided updates at the ICD-9-CM Coordination and Maintenance Committee meetings, which offered an opportunity for the public to provide feedback. The system developers have routinely maintained and updated the systems to keep pace with changing industry needs and trends. ICD-10-CM/PCS are publicly available on the NCHS and CMS Web sites, respectively.

Reasons for Implementation

ICD-10-CM/PCS represents a significant improvement over ICD-9-CM. Both ICD-10-CM and ICD-10-PCS were designed to overcome the problems and limitations in the ICD-9-CM system, bringing us more up to date by providing specific codes for conditions and procedures and providing more flexibility in adding new codes to the system. The new code sets incorporate much greater specificity and clinical detail, which would result in major improvements in the quality and usefulness of coded data. Medical terminology and the classification of diseases have been updated to be consistent with current clinical practice. Both ICD-10-CM and ICD-10-PCS have an improved structure and capacity for capturing technological advances. These systems are more flexible and able to accommodate revisions necessitated by medical advances.

The new codes have the potential to provide better data for evaluating and improving the quality of patient care. For example, data captured by the code sets could be used in more meaningful ways to better understand complications, design clinically robust algorithms, and track care outcomes.

Adoption of ICD-10-CM also would facilitate international comparisons of quality of care and the sharing of best practices globally.

Use of ICD-10-CM will standardize the reporting of public health information (including disease outbreaks and bioterrorism events) across the globe, achieve international health data comparability, and enable international comparisons of quality of care and sharing of best practices among different countries, since much of the rest of the world has already implemented ICD-10 or a clinical modification of this system.

ICD-10-CM/PCS is more amenable to the use of computer-assisted coding technology, which is expected to reduce the administrative costs associated with the current labor-intensive manual coding process and improve coding accuracy and consistency.

Emerging healthcare technologies and the need for interoperability amid the increase in adoption of electronic health records (EHRs) and personal health records (PHRs) require a standard code set that is expandable and sufficiently detailed to enable the accurate capture of current and future healthcare information. The implementation of ICD-10-CM/PCS will promote the use of health information technology and increase the overall value of EHRs.

The upgrade to the ICD-10-CM/PCS code sets offers providers and payers better data in support of their efforts to improve performance, create efficiencies, and contain costs. Greater specificity regarding clinical conditions and services delivered will provide payers, policy makers, and providers with better information to make major refinements to U.S. reimbursement systems, including the design and implementation of pay-for-performance programs. The use of ICD-10-CM/ PCS may also help reduce the opportunities for fraud and improve fraud detection capabilities, due to reduced coding ambiguity and misinterpretation.

Up-to-date classification systems will provide much better data for:

- Measuring the quality, safety, and efficacy of care
- Designing payment systems and processing claims for reimbursement
- Conducting research, epidemiological studies, and clinical trials
- Setting health policy
- Operational and strategic planning and designing healthcare delivery systems
- Monitoring resource utilization
- Improving clinical, financial, and administrative performance
- Preventing and detecting healthcare fraud and abuse
- Tracking public health and risks

It is anticipated that implementation of ICD-10-CM/PCS will improve administrative efficiencies and lower costs through:

- Increased use of automated tools to facilitate the coding process
- Decreased claims-associated submissions (attachments and request for additional

information) and claims adjudication costs
- Increased information that can justify quality and outcomes assessment
- Fewer rejected and improper reimbursement claims
- Decreased need for manual medical record documentation review
- Increased specificity in the area of disease and medical practice that cannot be described currently with ICD-9-CM codes
- Reduced coding errors
- Reduced labor costs and increased productivity

Extensive development and evaluation of ICD-10-CM/PCS as replacements for ICD-9-CM have been conducted. This includes system testing, completion of a comprehensive cost/benefit analysis, and hundreds of hours of testimony by experts who examined all sides of the issue. While the change-over to ICD-10-CM/PCS will have a major impact on the entire U.S. healthcare industry, a cost/benefit analysis conducted by the RAND Corporation for the NCVHS concluded that benefits of ICD-10-CM/PCS are likely to exceed initial implementation costs within just a few years.

Rulemaking Process

On August 22, 2008, HHS published a notice of proposed rulemaking (NPRM) for the adoption of ICD-10-CM/PCS code sets to replace the currently used ICD-9-CM code sets under rules 45 CFR Parts 160 and 162 of HIPAA. The *proposed* compliance date in the NPRM was October 1, 2011.

According to the proposed rule, HHS considered a number of alternatives to the adoption of the ICD-10 code sets. First, they considered extending the life of ICD-9-CM by assigning codes to new diagnoses and procedures without regard to the hierarchy of the code set. However, this approach does not represent a long-term solution to the code shortage, it does not address all of the shortcomings of ICD-9-CM, and it would destroy the natural hierarchy inherent in the code set. Current Procedural Terminology (CPT) ® was considered as a replacement for the ICD-9-CM procedure code set. However, a study undertaken by the Government Accountability Office (GAO) on the use of multiple procedure coding systems concluded that CPT® does not meet all of the criteria for standard code sets under HIPAA and the procedural code set requirements recommended by NCVHS. The GAO report stated that CPT® has not been shown to be acceptable or comprehensive enough to serve as a single procedure code set for reporting both hospital inpatient and outpatient physician services. Another option that was considered was to forego adoption of ICD-10 and wait until ICD-11 is ready. However, there are no firm timeframes for the completion of developmental work or testing and no firm implementation date has been designated. The earliest projected date for implementation would be 2020, assuming that no clinical modification is needed. Also, since ICD-11 will build upon ICD-10, many of the costs and much of the work associated with upgrading to ICD-11 will be mitigated by ICD-10 implementation.

After considering the various alternatives to replacing ICD-9-CM with ICD-10-CM/PCS, HHS concluded that adopting ICD-10-CM/PCS is the only viable alternative that would meet the long-term coding needs of the healthcare industry. The changeover to ICD-10-CM/PCS codes will have a major impact on the entire healthcare industry. However, HHS concluded that in the long-term, the benefits of ICD-10-CM/PCS outweigh the costs.

Final Rule Published

On January 16, 2009, HHS published the final rule adopting ICD-10-CM/PCS as replacements for the ICD-9-CM code set. The final compliance date is October 1, 2013. In establishing the compliance date, HHS sought to select a date that achieves a balance between the industry's need to implement ICD-10-CM/PCS within a feasible amount of time, and HHS' need to begin reaping the benefits of the use of these code sets; stop the hierarchical deterioration and other problems associated with the continued use of the ICD-9-CM code sets; align with the rest of the world's use of ICD-10 to achieve global health care data compatibility; plan and budget for the transition to ICD-10-CM/PCS appropriately; and mitigate the cost of further delays. HHS believes that an October 1, 2013 ICD-10-CM/PCS compliance date achieves that balance.

Effective Dates

Effective with encounter and discharge dates on or after October 1, 2013, the ICD-9-CM diagnosis code set will be replaced with ICD-10-CM (including the *ICD-10-CM Official Guidelines for Coding and Reporting*) for coding diseases, injuries, impairments, other health problems and their manifestations, and causes of injury, disease and impairment, or other health problems. The ICD-9-CM procedure code set will be replaced with ICD-10-PCS (including the *ICD-10-PCS Official Guidelines for Coding and Reporting*) for the following procedures or other actions taken for diseases, injuries and impairments on hospital inpatients reported by hospitals: prevention, diagnosis, treatment, and management.

ICD-10-CM/PCS Uses

ICD-10-CM will be used in all healthcare settings, whereas ICD-10-PCS will only be used for facility reporting of hospital inpatient services. CPT® and HCPCS Level II will continue to be used for reporting physician and other professional services and procedures performed in hospital outpatient departments and other outpatient facilities. ICD-9-CM codes, and not ICD-10-CM/PCS codes, will be used for all encounter and discharge dates prior to October 1, 2013. For example, a hospitalization with an admission date of September 20, 2013 and a discharge date of October 1, 2013 would be coded using the ICD-10-CM/PCS code sets, whereas a hospitalization with a discharge date of September 30, 2013 would be coded using the ICD-9-CM code set. HHS concluded that it would be in the health care industry's best interests if all entities were to comply with the ICD-10-CM/PCS code set standards at the same time to ensure the accuracy and timeliness of claims and transaction processing. A single compliance date will reduce the burden on both providers and insurers who will be able to edit on a single new coding system for claims received for encounters and discharges occurring on or after October 1, 2013.

The three key issues HHS believes necessitate the need to update from ICD-9-CM to ICD-10-CM/PCS are:

- ICD-9-CM is out of date and running out of space for new codes.
- ICD-10 is the international standard to report and monitor diseases and mortality, making it important for the United States to adopt ICD-10-based classifications for reporting and surveillance.
- ICD codes are core elements of many health information technology (HIT) systems, making the conversion to ICD-10-CM/PCS necessary to fully realize benefits of HIT adoption.

Implementation Issues
HHS anticipates that the use of ICD-10-CM, with its greater detail and granularity, will greatly enhance their capability to measure quality outcomes. The greater detail and granularity of ICD-10-CM/PCS will also provide more precision for claims- and value-based purchasing initiatives such as the hospital-acquired conditions (HAC) payment policy.

HHS does not anticipate that there will be any immediate changes to reimbursement with the initial implementation of ICD-10-CM/PCS. Data drives changes in reimbursement, and this data likely will not be available for quite some time after implementation, thus reimbursement changes will be accomplished on an incremental basis.

Updates to ICD

Changes and updates to ICD-9-CM are managed by the ICD-9-CM Coordination and Maintenance (C&M) Committee, a federal committee established in 1985 and co-chaired by representatives from NCHS and CMS. The committee is responsible for ongoing maintenance of ICD-9-CM. Although the ICD-9-CM C&M Committee is a federal committee, suggestions for modifications come from both the public and private sectors. Recommendations and comments are carefully reviewed and evaluated before any final decisions are made. No decisions are made at the meetings. The ICD-9-CM C&M Committee's role is advisory. All final decisions are made by the director of NCHS and the Administrator of CMS. This committee will be re-named the ICD-10 Coordination and Maintenance Committee at the time of implementation of ICD-10-CM/PCS and will be responsible for ongoing maintenance of these code sets. Until that time, ICD-10-CM/PCS is updated annually by NCHS and CMS, respectively. These updates reflect changes that have been made to ICD-9-CM as well as suggested modifications from the healthcare industry.

Version 5010

On January 16, 2009, HHS also published the final rule for adoption of the updated X12 standard, Version 5010, and the National Council for Prescription Drug Programs standard, Version D.0, for electronic transactions, such as healthcare claims. The updated version of the electronic transaction standards (version 5010) must be adopted before the ICD-10-CM/PCS code sets because the current version, version 4010, lacks the means to identify the code set being used on the claim. Version 5010 has anticipated the transition to ICD-10-CM/PCS by adding a qualifier so that the code set being used can be identified. The compliance date for implementation of version 5010 is January 1, 2012.

Chapter 2
ICD-10-CM

The ICD-10-CM code set is the U.S. clinical modification of the WHO's ICD-10 diagnosis classification system. It was developed by the National Center for Health Statistics (NCHS) in the Centers for Disease Control and Prevention (CDC), following a voluntary consensus-based process and working closely with specialty societies to ensure clinical utility and subject matter expert input into the process of creating the clinical modification, with comments from a number of medical specialty societies and organizations that addressed specific concerns or perceived unmet clinical needs encountered with ICD-9-CM. The NCHS also had discussions with other users, including nursing, rehabilitation, primary care providers, the National Committee for Quality Assurance, long-term and home health care providers, and managed care organizations to solicit their comments about ICD-10-CM. The NCHS has worked closely with many organizations to address the clinical needs in the United States to incorporate the level of detail needed in a morbidity classification and to provide code titles and language that complement accepted clinical practice for all users in the United States.

ICD-10-CM Enhancements

The ICD-10-CM code set provides much more information and detail within the codes than ICD-9-CM, facilitating timely electronic processing of claims by reducing requests for additional information. ICD-10-CM also includes significant improvements over ICD-9-CM in coding primary care encounters, external causes of injury, mental disorders, neoplasms, and preventive health. The ICD-10-CM code set reflects advances in medicine and medical technology, as well as accommodates the capture of more detail on socioeconomics, ambulatory care conditions, problems related to lifestyle, and the results of screening tests. It also provides for more space to accommodate future expansions, laterality for specifying which organ or part of the body is involved, as well as expanded distinctions for ambulatory and managed care encounters.

ICD-10-CM Format

The tenth revision has implemented a completely alphanumeric coding scheme. The first character is a letter. All the letters of the alphabet are used with the exception of the letter *U*, which has been set aside by WHO for the provisional assignment of new diseases of uncertain etiology (U00–U49) or for Bacterial agents resistant to antibiotics (U80–U89). ICD-10-CM has an index and tabular list similar to those of ICD-9-CM. ICD-10-CM consists of an alphabetic index formatted by main terms listed in alphabetic order with indentations for any applicable qualifiers or descriptors. Familiar punctuation such as brackets, parentheses, colons, and commas are used in ICD-10-CM, as are terms such as "Not Elsewhere Classified (NEC)," "Not Otherwise Specified (NOS)," "code first," "Use additional code," and "code also" notes familiar to coding professionals. Cross references are included to provide instructions to reference other or additional terms. The tabular list (table 2.1) is presented in code number order and used like ICD-9-CM.

Comparing ICD-9-CM and ICD-10-CM

ICD-10-CM differs from ICD-9-CM in its organization and structure, code composition, and level of detail. There are approximately 68,000 codes in ICD-10-CM and 14,000 codes in the ICD-9-CM diagnosis classification.

The letters *I* and *O* are used in ICD-10-CM, but they shouldn't be confused with the numbers 1 and 0 because the letters *I* and *O* are only used in the first character position and this character is always a letter.

Table 2.1. Tabular List

ICD-9-CM	ICD-10-CM
• Consists of three to five characters • First digit is numeric or alpha (*E* or *V*) • Second, third, fourth, and fifth digits are numeric • Always at least three digits • Decimal placed after the first three characters • Alpha characters are not case-sensitive	• Consists of three to seven characters • First character is alpha • All letters used except *U* • Second character is numeric • Characters 3–7 can be alpha or numeric • Decimal placed after the first three characters • Alpha characters are not case-sensitive

Familiar Hierarchy
ICD-10-CM has the same hierarchical structure as ICD-9-CM, and all codes with the same first three characters have common traits. Each character beyond the first three adds more specificity. Even though ICD-10-CM has more characters (up to seven) and uses alpha characters, each code must be at least three characters, with a decimal point used after the third character. Most, but not all, three-character categories have been subdivided. Up to four characters may follow the decimal. However, not every code will have four characters after the decimal; the concept is the same as ICD-9-CM.

Code Structure
The first character of the ICD-10-CM code is an alpha character, and each letter is associated with a particular chapter, except for the letters *D* and *H*. The letter *D* is used in both chapter 2, Neoplasms, and chapter 3, Diseases of the blood and blood-forming organs and certain disorders involving the immune mechanism. The letter *H* is used in both chapters 7, Diseases of the eye and adnexa, and 8, Diseases of the ear and mastoid process. To allow for future revisions or expansions of the classification, every available code is not used. See figure 2.1.

Figure 2.1. Code structure of ICD-10-CM versus ICD-9-CM

ICD-10-CM codes may consist of up to seven characters.

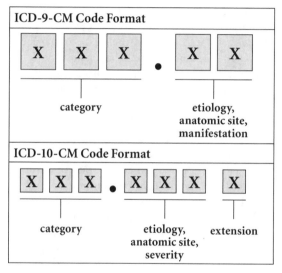

ICD-10-CM also has the same use of notes and instructions as ICD-9-CM. When a note appears under a three-character code, it applies to all codes within that category, and notes under a specific code apply to the single code. ICD-10-CM and ICD-9-CM also have many of the same conventions and guidelines.

Changes in ICD-10-CM

The principal changes in ICD-10-CM are in its organization and structure, code composition, and level of detail. Changes in the ICD-10-CM code set include the following (changes specific to a particular chapter are described under the relevant chapter in Chapter-Specific Changes section below):

- ICD-10-CM consists of 21 chapters.
- The order of some chapters has been rearranged.
- A sixth character has been added in some chapters.
- A seventh character has been added in some chapters (primarily in the Pregnancy, Injury, and External Cause chapters).
- ICD-10-CM includes full code titles for all codes (no references back to common fourth and fifth digits).
- The codes corresponding to ICD-9-CM V codes (Factors Influencing Health Status and Contact with Health Services) and E codes (External Causes of Injury and Poisoning) are incorporated into the main classification and are not separated into supplementary classifications as they were in ICD-9-CM.
- Conditions with newly discovered etiology or treatment protocols have been reclassified to a more appropriate chapter.
- The codes for postoperative complications have been expanded and a distinction made between intraoperative complications and postprocedural disorders.
- Many postoperative complications have been moved to the appropriate procedure-specific

body system chapter.
- Category restructuring and code reorganization have occurred in a number of ICD-10-CM chapters, which has resulted in the classification of certain diseases and disorders differently from the ninth revision.
- A dummy placeholder x is used in some codes to allow for future expansion and also to fill out empty characters when a code contains fewer than six characters and a seventh character extension applies.
- In some cases, instructional notes indicate a change in code sequencing from ICD-9-CM (for example, for anemia in neoplastic disease, an instructional note indicates that the neoplasm should be coded first).
- Instructional notes indicating that an additional code should be assigned for an associated condition or that an underlying condition should be coded first have been expanded.
- A number of combination codes for conditions and common symptoms or manifestations have been added.
- Laterality (meaning left or right side) has been added where applicable.
- Extensions have been added for type of encounter (initial, subsequent, and sequela) for injuries and external causes.
- Changes have been made in the timeframes specified in certain codes.
- Detail relevant to ambulatory and managed care encounters has been expanded.

New Features
Combination Codes
The use of combination codes solves many of
the sequencing dilemmas currently encountered
with the use of ICD-9-CM. ICD-10-CM includes
combination codes for conditions and common
symptoms or manifestations. A single code may be
used to classify two diagnoses, a diagnosis with an
associated sign or symptom, or a diagnosis with an
associated complication. This allows one code to be
assigned, resulting in fewer cases requiring more
than one code and reducing sequencing problems.
Combination codes are also available for external
causes and poisonings, with information combined
into one code (including the drug involved).

Laterality
ICD-10-CM includes codes for laterality (unclassi-
fied in ICD-9-CM). Codes for left side, right side,
and in some cases, bilateral are available in applicable chapters. If the side is not documented in
the medical record, a code for "unspecified side"
is available. If no bilateral code is provided and the
condition is bilateral, assign separate codes for both
the left and right side. The majority of codes affected
by laterality are in the neoplasm and injury chapters.

Excludes Notes
ICD-10-CM also includes added standard definitions for two types of excludes notes. Excludes1
indicates *not coded here*. The code being excluded
is never used with the code. The two conditions
cannot occur together. For example, B06 Rubella

[German measles] has an Excludes1 of congenital rubella (P35.0).

Excludes2 indicates *not included here.* The excluded condition is not part of the condition represented by the code. It is acceptable to use both codes together if the patient has both conditions. For example, J04.0, Acute laryngitis has an Excludes2 of chronic laryngitis (J37.0).

Other Changes

Expanded codes are available in many sections of ICD-10-CM, particularly in the injury, diabetes, alcohol and substance abuse, and postoperative complication sections.

The following chapters have undergone significant revision: Chapter 5, Mental and Behavioral Disorders; Chapter 19, Injury, Poisoning, and Certain Other Consequences of External Causes; and Chapter 20, External Causes of Morbidity.

The codes for postoperative complications include a distinction between intraoperative complications and postprocedural disorders. ICD-10-CM provides 50 different codes for "complications of foreign body accidentally left in body following a procedure," compared to only one code in ICD-9-CM.

Newly recognized conditions and conditions not uniquely identified in ICD-9-CM have been given codes, such as subsequent myocardial infarction and mesothelioma. Conditions with a recently-discovered etiology or new treatment protocol have been reassigned to a more appropriate chapter. For example, gout has been reassigned to the musculoskeletal chapter in ICD-10-CM (it was in the

Endocrine chapter in ICD-9-CM).

It is important to note that sometimes distinctions made in ICD-9-CM codes are not included in ICD-10-CM because they are no longer considered important or clinically relevant. For example, the ICD-10-CM tuberculosis codes no longer specify the method by which the disease was confirmed (bacteriological or histological examination).

Although specificity and detail have been significantly expanded in ICD-10-CM, there are still non-specific codes available when there is no information to support a more specific code.

Seventh Character Code Extensions

Seventh character code extensions have been added in some chapters, primarily in the obstetrics, injury, and external cause chapters. They may be either alpha or numeric and are added to the end of the code in the seventh position when applicable. They provide additional information about the characteristics of the encounter. Extensions have different meanings depending on the section. A code that has an applicable 7th character is considered invalid without the 7th character.

Official Guidelines for Coding and Reporting

As with ICD-9-CM, proper coding relies on use of the official coding guidelines. The *ICD-10-CM Official Guidelines for Coding and Reporting* contain all information about the coding conventions for ICD-10-CM, general use guidelines, and chapter-specific guidelines. The purpose of the guidelines is to assist users in coding and reporting in situations where ICD9CM does not provide direction. The official coding guidelines apply to the proper use of ICD-9-CM, regardless of the healthcare setting. The guidelines for coding and reporting have been developed and approved by the Cooperating Parties. The Cooperating Parties are the American Hospital Association (AHA), the AHIMA, CMS, and NCHS. Coding and sequencing instructions in ICD-9-CM take precedence over any guidelines.

New or revised guidelines pertaining to a specific ICD-10-CM chapter are included in the chapter-specific changes below.

Chapter-Specific Changes in ICD-10-CM

Some of the key chapter-specific changes in ICD-10-CM are highlighted below, note that is not possible to list every change from ICD-9-CM.

Chapter 1: Infectious and Parasitic Diseases (A00–B99)

Some codes have been moved from another chapter in ICD-9-CM to chapter 1 in ICD-10-CM. For example, the code for tetanus neonatorum has been moved from ICD-9-CM chapter 15, Certain Conditions Originating in the Perinatal Period to ICD-10-CM chapter 1. Also, obstetrical tetanus has been moved from category 670 in the obstetrics chapter of ICD-9-CM to category A34 in chapter 1 of ICD-10-CM.

Chapter 1 of ICD-10-CM includes a new section called "Infections with a predominantly sexual mode of transmission (A50–A64)." Many codes have been moved into this section from other places in the ICD-9-CM classification.

Chapter 2: Neoplasms (C00–D49)

Some codes have moved to chapter 2 from other chapters. For example, Waldenstrom's macroglobulinemia is classified to category 273, Disorders of plasma protein metabolism in ICD-9-CM chapter 3, Endocrine, Nutritional and Metabolic Diseases and Immunity Disorders, but it is classified to category C88, Malignant immunoproliferative diseases, in chapter 2, Neoplasms, in ICD-10-CM.

Also, the classification of malignant neoplasms of the retroperitoneum and peritoneum falls within the subchapter titled "Malignant neoplasms of digestive organs and peritoneum" in ICD-9-CM, whereas these codes are located in a section titled "Malignant neoplasms of mesothelial and soft tissue" in ICD-10-CM.

Melanoma in situ has a unique category, D03. In ICD-9-CM, melanoma in situ is included in category 172, Malignant melanoma of skin.

Chapter 3: Diseases of the Blood and Blood-Forming Organs and Certain Disorders Involving the Immune Mechanism (D50–D89)

Chapter 3 of ICD-10-CM includes codes primarily from ICD-9-CM chapter 4, Diseases of the Blood and Blood-Forming Organs, but also includes many codes from ICD-9-CM chapter 3, Endocrine, Nutritional and Metabolic Diseases and Immunity Disorders. It also includes some codes from ICD-9-CM chapter 1, Infectious and Parasitic Diseases (for example, sarcoidosis).

Chapter 4: Endocrine, Nutritional, and Metabolic Diseases (E00–E90)

The diabetes mellitus codes are combination codes that include the type of diabetes, the body system affected, and the complications affecting that body system. As many diabetes codes as are necessary to describe all of the complications of the disease may be used. They should be sequenced based on the reason for a particular encounter.

The category for diabetes mellitus has been updated to reflect the current clinical classification of diabetes.

The diabetes mellitus codes are no longer distinguished as controlled or uncontrolled.

Chapter 5: Mental and Behavioral Disorders (F01–F99)

The arrangement of the codes within the various sections is significantly different.

A number of changes to category and subcategory titles have been made. For example, ICD-9-CM subcategory 296.0 is titled "Bipolar I disorder, single manic episode," whereas the ICD-10-CM counterpart, category F30, is titled "Manic episode."

There are unique codes for alcohol and drug use not specified as abuse or dependence.

Codes for drug and alcohol abuse and dependence no longer identify continuous or episodic use.

There are combination codes for drug and alcohol use and associated conditions, such as withdrawal, sleep disorders, or psychosis.

There is a change in sequencing involving the mental retardation codes. In ICD-9-CM, an additional code for any associated psychiatric or physical condition(s) should be sequenced after the mental retardation code. In ICD-10-CM, any associated physical or developmental disorder should be coded first.

Chapter 6: Diseases of the Nervous System (G00–G99)

Sense organs have been separated from nervous system disorders, creating two new chapters for Diseases of Eye and Adnexa and Diseases of the Ear and Mastoid Process.

Basilar and carotid artery syndromes, transient global amnesia, and transient cerebral ischemic attack have been moved from ICD-9-CM chapter 7, Diseases of the Circulatory System, to ICD-10-CM chapter 6.

Chapter 7: Diseases of the Eye and Adnexa (H00–H59)

Chapter 7 is an entirely new chapter in ICD-10-CM. In ICD-9-CM, these conditions were classified to chapter 6, Diseases of the Nervous System and Sense Organs.

The term "senile" is not used in ICD-10-CM to describe a type of cataract; the term "age-related" is used instead.

Codes have been expanded to increase anatomic specificity and add the concept of laterality.

Chapter 8: Diseases of the Ear and Mastoid Process (H60–H95)

Chapter 8 is also a new chapter in ICD-10-CM. It encompasses conditions that are classified to ICD-9-CM chapter 6, Diseases of the Nervous System and Sense Organs.

Codes have been expanded to increase anatomic specificity and add the concept of laterality.

A number of new instructional notes indicating that the underlying disease should be coded first have been added. For example, there is a note under the ICD-10-CM category for perforation of tympanic membrane indicating that any associated otitis media should be coded first.

Chapter 9: Diseases of the Circulatory System (I00–I99)

Some codes have been moved to this chapter from other chapters in ICD-9-CM. For example, Binswanger's disease has been moved from ICD-9-CM chapter 5, Mental Disorders, to ICD-10-CM chapter 9.

Codes for chronic and mesenteric lymphadenitis have moved to this chapter from ICD-9-CM chapter 4, Diseases of the Blood and Blood-Forming Organs.

Gangrene has moved to this chapter from ICD-9-CM chapter 16, Symptoms, Signs, and Ill-Defined Conditions.

The category for late effects of cerebrovascular disease has been retitled "Sequelae of cerebrovascular disease," and it has been restructured by expanding all subcategory codes. This expansion involves specifying laterality, changing subcategory titles, making terminology changes, adding sixth characters, and providing greater specificity in general. Late effects of cerebrovascular disease are differentiated by type of stroke (hemorrhage, infarction).

The terminology used to describe some cardiovascular conditions in ICD-10-CM is different than the terms used in ICD-9-CM. For example, "intermediate coronary syndrome" has been retitled "unstable angina."

In the acute myocardial infarction codes, ST elevation (STEMI) and non-ST-elevation (NSTEMI) are in the ICD-10-CM code titles instead of just being inclusion terms.

The time frame for use of the acute myocardial infarction (AMI) codes has changed from eight weeks or less in ICD-9-CM to four weeks or less in ICD-10-CM.

Chapter 9 contains codes for subsequent AMIs. A code from category I22, Subsequent ST elevation (STEMI) and non ST elevation (NSTEMI) myocardial infarction, is to be used when a patient who has suffered an AMI has a new AMI within the four week time frame of the initial AMI. A code from category I22 must be used in conjunction with a code from category I21, ST elevation (STEMI) and non-ST elevation (NSTEMI) myocardial infarction. The sequencing of the I21 and I22 codes depends on the circumstances of the encounter.

The type of hypertension (benign, malignant, or unspecified) is not used as an axis for the ICD-10-CM hypertension codes.

Chapter 10: Diseases of the Respiratory System (J00–J99)

Certain codes have moved to chapter 10. For example, streptococcal sore throat is in chapter 1, Infectious and Parasitic Diseases, in ICD-9-CM, whereas it is in chapter 10 in ICD-10-CM.

Lobar pneumonia is no longer classified to the code for pneumococcal pneumonia. It has a unique code in a category for pneumonia, unspecified organism.

The terminology used to describe asthma has been updated to reflect the current clinical classification of asthma. Instead of asthma being described as extrinsic or intrinsic, it is classified as mild intermittent, mild persistent, moderate persistent, and severe persistent.

Some of the codes in chapter 10 have been expanded to include notes indicating that an additional code should be assigned or an associated condition should be sequenced first. There are four types of this category of instructional notes in chapter 10:

1. Use additional code to identify the infectious agent
2. Use additional code to identify the virus
3. Code first any associated lung abscess
4. Code first the underlying disease

Chapter 11: Diseases of the Digestive System (K00–K94)

Some codes have been moved from other chapters in ICD-9-CM to chapter 11 in ICD-10-CM. For example, angiodysplasia of intestine is in a subcategory for "other specified disorders of intestine" in ICD-9-CM, whereas it is in a subcategory for "vascular disorders of intestine" in ICD-10-CM.

Some of the disease categories in chapter 11 have been restructured to bring together those groups that are in some way related. For example, chapter 11 contains two new sections: Diseases of liver (K70–K77) and Disorders of gallbladder, biliary tract, and pancreas (K80–K87).

Instructional notes indicating that an additional code should be assigned for associated conditions and external causes or that an underlying condition should be coded first have been expanded.

Chapter 12: Diseases of the Skin and Subcutaneous Tissue (L00–L99)

Chapter 12 has been completely re-structured to bring together groups of diseases that are related to one another in some way. The corresponding ICD-9-CM chapter contains only three subsections, whereas chapter 12 in ICD-10-CM contains nine subsections (often referred to as "blocks" in ICD-10-CM).

Instructional notes have been expanded indicating that an additional code should be used to identify the organism or that the drug or substance, underlying disease, or associated underlying condition should be coded first.

A note under block L20–L30, Dermatitis and eczema, indicates that in this block, the terms "dermatitis" and "eczema" are used synonymously and interchangeably.

For pressure ulcers, the site, laterality, and severity are specified in a single code in ICD-10-CM. Any associated gangrene should be sequenced first.

Chapter 13: Diseases of the Musculoskeletal System and Connective Tissue (M00–M99)

A number of block, category, and subcategory title changes have been made in chapter 13. For example, ICD-9-CM subsection 710–719 is titled "Arthropathies and related disorders," whereas the corresponding section in ICD-10-CM, M00–M25, is titled "Arthropathies."

A number of conditions have moved to chapter 13 from other chapters in ICD-9-CM. For example, gout is classified to ICD-9-CM chapter 3, Endocrine, Nutritional, and Metabolic Diseases, and Immunity Disorders, whereas it is classified to chapter 13 in ICD-10-CM.

Polyarteritis nodosa has moved to this chapter from ICD-9-CM chapter 7, Diseases of the Circulatory System.

ICD-9-CM categories 524, Dentofacial anomalies, including malocclusion, and 526, Diseases of the jaw, have been moved from ICD-9-CM chapter 9, Diseases of the Digestive System, to ICD-10-CM chapter 13.

Bone, joint, or muscle conditions that are the result of a healed injury are usually found in chapter 13. Recurrent bone, joint, or muscle conditions are also usually found in chapter 13. Any current, acute injury should be coded to the appropriate injury code from chapter 19, Injury, Poisoning, and Certain Other Consequences of External Causes. Chronic or recurrent conditions should generally be coded with a code from chapter 13.

Almost every code in chapter 13 has been greatly expanded in some way. In many cases, this expansion includes greater anatomic specificity and laterality.

The following 7th character extensions are required for codes in chapter 13 that represent pathological or stress fractures:

A – Initial encounter for fracture

D – Subsequent encounter for fracture with routine healing

G – Subsequent encounter for fracture with delayed healing

K – Subsequent encounter for fracture with nonunion

P – Subsequent encounter for fracture with
    malunion
S – Sequela

Seventh character A is for use as long as the patient is receiving active treatment for the fracture. Examples of active treatment are: surgical treatment, emergency department encounter, evaluation, and treatment by a new physician. Seventh character D is to be used for encounters after the patient has completed active treatment.

As with many of the other chapters, instructional notes have been expanded indicating that additional codes should be assigned for associated conditions or an underlying condition should be coded first.

Chapter 14: Diseases of the Genitourinary System (N00–N99)

A number of block and category title changes have been made in chapter 14. For example, ICD-9-CM subsection 617–629 is titled "Other disorders of female genital tract," whereas the corresponding section in ICD-10-CM, N80–N98, is titled "Noninflammatory disorders of female genital tract."

Some codes that were in other chapters in ICD-9-CM have been moved to chapter 14. For example, ICD-9-CM code 099.40, Other nongonococcal urethritis, unspecified, is in ICD-9-CM chapter 1, Infectious and Parasitic Diseases, but its ICD-10-CM counterpart, code N34.1, Nonspecific urethritis, is in chapter 14 in ICD-10-CM.

Chapter 15: Pregnancy, Childbirth and the Puerperium (O00–O9A)

Some codes have been moved from other chapters in ICD-9-CM to chapter 15 in ICD-10-CM. For example, encounter for supervision of high-risk pregnancy has been moved from the ICD-9-CM Supplementary Classification of Factors Influencing Health Status and Contact with Health Services to ICD-10-CM chapter 15.

The codes in chapter 15 identify the trimester in which the condition occurred rather than the episode of care (delivered, antepartum, or postpartum) identified in the ICD-9-CM obstetric codes. Because certain obstetric conditions or complications occur during certain trimesters, not all conditions include codes for all three trimesters. And some codes do not include a character to describe the trimester at all because the condition always occurs in a specific trimester, or the concept of trimester of pregnancy is not applicable.

The time frame for differentiating the abortion and fetal death codes has changed from 22 to 20 weeks.

The time frame for differentiating early and late vomiting in pregnancy has been changed from 22 to 20 weeks.

Certain codes in chapter 15 require a 7th character extension to identify the fetus in a multiple gestation that is affected by the condition being coded. These are the applicable 7th character extensions:

0 – not applicable or unspecified
1 – fetus 1
2 – fetus 2
3 – fetus 3
4 – fetus 4
5 – fetus 5
9 – other fetus

The 7th character "0" is for single gestations and multiple gestations where the affected fetus is unspecified.

Chapter 16: Certain Conditions Originating in the Perinatal Period (P00–P96)

A number of block and category title changes have been made in chapter 16. For example, ICD-9-CM subsection 760–763 is titled "Maternal causes of perinatal morbidity and mortality," whereas the ICD-10-CM counterpart, P00–P04, is titled "Newborn affected by maternal factors and by complications of pregnancy, labor, and delivery."

The phrase "fetus or newborn" used in many ICD-9-CM codes is not used in ICD-10-CM. The term "newborn" is consistently used in code titles in chapter 16 to clarify that these codes are for use on newborn records only, never on maternal records.

Chapter 17: Congenital Malformations, Deformations, and Chromosomal Abnormalities (Q00–Q99)

A number of block, category, subcategory, and code title changes have been made in chapter 17. For example, in ICD-9-CM, code 758.1 is titled "Patau's syndrome," whereas the counterpart codes in ICD-10-CM are titled "Trisomy 13."

Many codes for congenital conditions and chromosomal abnormalities have been expanded in ICD-10-CM. For example, in ICD-9-CM, chromosomal anomalies are classified to category 758. In ICD-10-CM, there are nine categories for chromosomal abnormalities, not elsewhere classified.

Chapter 18: Symptoms, Signs, and Abnormal Clinical and Laboratory Findings, Not Elsewhere Classified (R00–R99)

Chapter 18 includes symptoms, signs, abnormal results of clinical or other investigative procedures, and ill-defined conditions regarding which no diagnosis classifiable elsewhere is recorded.

The codes included in chapter 18 are limited to signs and symptoms that are not otherwise specified, of unknown etiology, or are transient. In general, categories in this chapter include the less well-defined conditions and symptoms that, without the necessary study to establish a final diagnosis, point to two or more diseases or body systems. Signs and symptoms that point to a diagnosis have been assigned to the appropriate body system chapter.

The conditions, signs, and symptoms included in chapter 18 consist of the following: cases for which no more specific diagnosis can be made even after all the facts bearing on the case have been investigated; signs or symptoms existing at the time of the initial encounter that proved to be transient and whose causes could not be determined; provisional diagnosis in a patient who failed to return for further investigation or care; cases referred elsewhere for investigation or treatment before the diagnosis was made; cases in which a more precise diagnosis was not available for any other reason; and certain symptoms, for which supplementary information is provided, that represent important problems in medical care in their own right.

Systemic inflammatory response syndrome (SIRS) is classified to category R65, Symptoms and signs specifically associated with systemic inflammation and infection. Codes in this category identify SIRS of noninfectious origin with and without acute organ dysfunction and severe sepsis with and without septic shock. An instructional note indicates that the underlying condition (or underlying infection, in the case of severe sepsis) should be coded first. Sepsis is not classified to category R65. Sepsis should be coded to the infection. For example, code A41.9 should be assigned for sepsis, unspecified.

Some codes that were in other chapters in ICD-9-CM have been moved to chapter 18. For example, bradycardia is classified to ICD-9-CM chapter 7, Diseases of the Circulatory System, and it is classified to chapter 18 in ICD-10-CM.

Pleurisy was classified to ICD-9-CM chapter 8, Diseases of the Respiratory System, but has been moved to chapter 18 in ICD-10-CM.

ICD-10-CM subcategory R40.2, Coma, incorporates the Glasgow coma scale (subcategories R40.21–R40.23). The Glasgow coma scale codes can be used in conjunction with traumatic brain injury or sequelae of cerebrovascular disease codes. They are primarily for use by trauma registries, but they may be used in any setting where this information is collected. The diagnosis code should be sequenced before the Glasgow coma scale codes. Three codes, one from each subcategory (R40.21, R40.22, and R40.23) are needed to complete the scale. The 7th character extension indicates when the scale was recorded, and it should match for all three codes:

0 – unspecified time

1 – in the field [EMT or ambulance]

2 – at arrival to emergency department

3 – at hospital admission

4 – 24 hours or more after hospital admission

Chapter 19: Injury, Poisoning, and Certain Other Consequences of External Causes (S00–T88)

Injuries are grouped by body part rather than by categories of injury, so that all injuries of the specific site (such as head and neck) are grouped together rather than groupings of all fractures or all open wounds. For example, categories in ICD-9-CM grouped by injury such as fractures (800–829), dislocations (830–839), and sprains and strains (840–848) are grouped in ICD-10-CM by site, such as injuries to the head (S00–S09), injuries to the neck (S10–S19), and injuries to the thorax (S20–S29).

The *S* section of chapter 19 provides codes for the various types of injuries related to single body regions. The *T* section covers injuries to unspecified body regions as well as poisonings and certain other consequences of external causes.

Certain codes, such as fractures, include much greater specificity in ICD-10-CM. For example, some of the information that may be found in fracture codes includes the type of fracture, specific anatomical site, whether the fracture is displaced or not, laterality, routine vs. delayed healing, nonunions, and malunions. Laterality and identification of type of encounter (initial, subsequent, sequela) are a significant component of the code expansion in chapter 19.

Fracture 7th character extensions include:

A – Initial encounter for closed fracture

B – Initial encounter for open fracture

D – Subsequent encounter for fracture with routine healing

G – Subsequent encounter for fracture with delayed healing

K – Subsequent encounter for fracture with nonunion

P – Subsequent encounter for fracture with malunion

S – Sequela

Some fracture categories provide for 7th character extensions to designate the specific type of open fracture (these designations are based on the

Gustilo open fracture classification):

 B – Initial encounter for open fracture type I or II (open NOS or not otherwise specified)

 C – Initial encounter for open fracture type IIIA, IIIB, or IIIC

 E – Subsequent encounter for open fracture type I or II with routine healing

 F – Subsequent encounter for open fracture type IIIA, IIIB, or IIIC with routine healing

 H – Subsequent encounter for open fracture type I or II with delayed healing

 J – Subsequent encounter for open fracture type IIIA, IIIB, or IIIC with delayed healing

 M – Subsequent encounter for open fracture type I or II with nonunion

 N – Subsequent encounter for open fracture type IIIA, IIIB, or IIIC with nonunion

 Q – Subsequent encounter for open fracture type I or II with malunion

 R – Subsequent encounter for open fracture type IIIA, IIIB, or IIIC with malunion

The extensions for "initial encounter" are used while the patient is receiving active treatment for the injury. Examples of active treatment are: surgical treatment, emergency department encounter, and evaluation and treatment by a new physician.

The extensions for "subsequent encounter" are used for encounters after the patient has received active treatment of the injury and is receiving routine care for the injury during the healing or recovery phase. Examples of subsequent care are:

cast change or removal, removal of external of internal fixation device, medication adjustment, and other aftercare and follow up visits following injury treatment.

Extension S, sequela, is for use for complications or conditions that arise as a direct result of an injury, such as scar formation after a burn. The scars are sequela of the burn. When using extension S, it is necessary to use both the injury code that precipitated the sequela and the code for the sequela itself. The S is added only to the injury code, not the sequela code. The S extension identifies the injury responsible for the sequela. The specific type of sequela (for example, scar) is sequenced first, followed by the injury code.

The aftercare Z codes should not be used for aftercare for injuries. For aftercare of an injury, assign the acute injury code with the appropriate 7th character for "subsequent encounter."

There are combination codes for poisonings and the associated external cause (accidental, intentional self-harm, assault, and undetermined).

Underdosing is a new concept in ICD-10-CM. Underdosing is taking less of a medication than is prescribed by a physician or the manufacturer's instruction, whether inadvertently or deliberately, with a resulting negative health consequence. A code for noncompliance (Z91.12-, Z91.13-) or failure in dosage during surgical or medical care (Y63.-) must be used with an underdosing code to indicate intent.

Chapter 20: External Causes of Morbidity (V00–Y98)

Chapter 20 permits the classification of environmental events and circumstances as the cause of injury, and other adverse effects. Where a code from this section is applicable, it is intended that it shall be used secondary to a code from another chapter of the Classification indicating the nature of the condition. Most often, the condition will be classifiable to Chapter 19, Injury, poisoning and certain other consequences of external causes (S00–T98). Other conditions that may be stated to be due to external causes are classified in Chapters 1 to 18. For these conditions, codes from Chapter 20 should be used to provide additional information as to the cause of the condition.

An external cause code may be used with any code in the range of A00.0–T88.9, Z00–Z99, classification that is a health condition due to an external cause. Though they are most applicable to injuries, they are also valid for use with such things as infections or diseases due to an external source, and other health conditions, such as a heart attack that occurs during strenuous physical activity.

Assign the external cause code, with the appropriate 7th character (initial encounter, subsequent encounter, or sequela) for each encounter for which the injury or condition is being treated.

In ICD-9-CM, the late effect codes for external causes are located in various subsections of the External Cause chapter. In ICD-10-CM, all late effects of external causes are identified by the addition of the 7th character extension S, Sequela, to the code for each intent (for example, accident or suicide).

Chapter 21: Factors Influencing Health Status and Contact with Health Services (Z00–Z99)

Certain codes have been moved from other chapters in ICD-9-CM to chapter 21 in ICD-10-CM. For example, elective, legal, or therapeutic abortions have been moved from ICD-9-CM chapter 11, Complications of Pregnancy, Childbirth, and the Puerperium, to ICD-10-CM chapter 21.

A number of codes have been expanded in chapter 21. For example, personal and family history codes have been expanded, including the addition of codes for personal history secondary malignant neoplasms.

Codes have been added for concepts that currently do not exist in ICD-9-CM. For example, code Z66 is to be used to indicate a "do not resuscitate" status. Category Z67 identifies the patient's blood type.

Note that there are also concepts that existed in ICD-9-CM that no longer exist in ICD-10-CM. For example, there is no comparable category in ICD-10-CM to ICD-9-CM category V57, Care involving use of rehabilitation procedures. For encounters for rehabilitative therapy, report the underlying condition for which therapy is being provided (such as an injury) with the appropriate 7th character extension indicating subsequent encounter.

ICD-10-CM consists of many new features and greater specificity. Code examples are provided in figure 2.2 to illustrate some of the differences between ICD-9-CM and ICD-10-CM.

Figure 2.2. ICD-9-CM and ICD-10-CM code comparisons—Examples

ICD-10-CM Code/Title	ICD-9-CM Code/Title	Key Difference(s) in ICD-10-CM
B27.01, Gammaherpesviral mononucleosis with polyneuropathy	075, Infectious mononucleosis	Specificity as to type of mononucleosis and associated complications
C50.211, Malignant neoplasm of upper-inner quadrant of right female breast	174.2, Malignant neoplasm of female breast, upper-inner quadrant	Laterality
D61.1, Drug-induced aplastic anemia	284.89, Other specified aplastic anemias	Specificity regarding cause
E10.331, Type 1 diabetes mellitus with moderate nonproliferative diabetic retinopathy with macular edema	250.51, Diabetes with ophthalmic manifestations, type 1, not stated as uncontrolled + 362.05, Moderate nonproliferative diabetic retinopathy + 362.07, Diabetic macular edema	Combination code for diabetes and associated complications; no identification of controlled vs. uncontrolled
F14.251, Cocaine dependence with cocaine-induced psychotic disorder with hallucinations	292.12, Drug-induced psychotic disorder with hallucinations + 304.20, Cocaine dependence, unspecified	Combination code for drug dependence and associated complications; no identification of whether drug use is continuous or episodic

ICD-10-CM Code/Title	ICD-9-CM Code/Title	Key Difference(s) in ICD-10-CM
G97.51, Postprocedural hemorrhage and hematoma of a nervous system organ or structure following a nervous system procedure	998.11, Hemorrhage complicating a procedure OR 998.12, Hematoma complicating a procedure	Distinction between intraoperative and postprocedural complications; many postoperative complications have been moved to body system chapters; hemorrhage and hematoma are included in single code
H35.353, Cystoid macular degeneration, bilateral	362.53, Cystoid macular degeneration	Laterality
H65.115, Acute and subacute allergic otitis media (mucoid) (sanguinous) (serous), recurrent, left ear	381.02, Acute mucoid otitis media OR 381.03, Acute sanguinous otitis media OR 381.04, Acute allergic serous otitis media OR 381.05, Acute allergic mucoid otitis media OR 381.06, Acute allergic sanguinous otitis media	Laterality; distinctions in ICD-9-CM not included in ICD-10-CM
I25.110, Arteriosclerotic heart disease of native coronary artery with unstable angina pectoris	414.01, Coronary atherosclerosis of native coronary artery + 411.1, Intermediate coronary syndrome	Combination code for underlying condition and associated manifestation; terminology change
I61.3, Nontraumatic intracerebral hemorrhage in brain stem	431, Intracerebral hemorrhage	Specificity

ICD-10-CM Code/Title	ICD-9-CM Code/Title	Key Difference(s) in ICD-10-CM
J20.1, Acute bronchitis due to Hemophilus influenzae	466.0, Acute bronchitis + 041.5, Bacterial infection in conditions classified elsewhere, Hemophilus influenza [H. influenza]	Combination code that includes both the disease and the organism
K50.113, Crohn's disease of large intestine with fistula	555.1, Regional enteritis of large intestine + 569.81, Fistula of intestine, excluding rectum and anus	Combination code that includes both the underlying disease and associated complications; terminology change
L02.213, Cutaneous abscess of chest wall	682.2, Other cellulitis and abscess, trunk	Specificity
M05.571, Rheumatoid polyneuropathy with rheumatoid arthritis of right ankle and foot	714.0, Rheumatoid arthritis + 357.1, Polyneuropathy in collagen vascular disease	Combination code that includes underlying condition and associated manifestation; site specificity
N03.6, Chronic nephritic syndrome with dense deposit disease	582.2, Chronic glomerulonephritis with lesion of membranoproliferative glomerulonephritis	Specificity; terminology change

ICD-10-CM Code/Title	ICD-9-CM Code/Title	Key Difference(s) in ICD-10-CM
O64.5xx2, Obstructed labor due to compound presentation, fetus 2	660.0x, Obstruction caused by malposition of fetus at onset of labor + 652.8x, Other specified malposition or malpresentation	Combination code that includes both the obstructed labor and the underlying cause; 7th character extension identifying that fetus 2 in a multiple gestation is the affected fetus; use of dummy placeholders (note that 5th digit in ICD-9-CM codes cannot be assigned without additional information as to the episode of care)
P12.4, Injury of scalp of newborn due to monitoring equipment	767.19, Birth trauma, Other injuries to scalp	Specificity
Q93.3, Deletion of short arm of chromosome 4	758.39, Other autosomal deletions	Specificity
R54, Age-related physical debility	797, Senility without mention of psychosis	Specificity; terminology change
S61.021A, Laceration with foreign body of right thumb without damage to nail, initial encounter	883.1, Open wound of fingers, complicated	Specificity; terminology change; laterality; type of encounter; type of complication identified instead of characterizing wound as "complicated"

ICD-10-CM Code/Title	ICD-9-CM Code/Title	Key Difference(s) in ICD-10-CM
S72.141D, Displaced intertrochanteric fracture of right femur, Subsequent encounter for closed fracture with routine healing	V54.13, Aftercare for healing traumatic fracture of hip	Specificity; type of encounter; different approach for classifying postacute encounters
T81.524S, Obstruction due to foreign body accidently left in body following endoscopic examination, Sequela	909.3, Late effect of complications of surgical and medical care	Specificity; type of encounter
T39.011A, Poisoning by aspirin, accidental (unintentional), Initial encounter	965.1, Poisoning by salicylates + E850.3, Accidental poisoning by salicylates	Combination code including poisoning and associated external cause; type of encounter
X39.01xA, Exposure to radon, Initial encounter	E926.8, Exposure to other specified radiation	Specificity; type of encounter
Z02.1, Encounter for pre-employment examination	V70.5, Health examination of defined subpopulations	Specificity

Chapter 3
ICD-10-Procedure Coding System (ICD-10-PCS)

Development of ICD-10-PCS

History

The procedure system of ICD-9-CM (volume 3) has been used in the United States to report inpatient procedures since 1979. Its structure has not permitted new procedures associated with rapidly changing technology to be effectively incorporated as new codes because of its limited capacity for expansion.

Development of ICD-10-PCS was funded by the Health Care Financing Administration (HCFA), now known as the Centers for Medicare & Medicaid Services (CMS), through a contract with 3M Health Information Systems. The system was under development for over five years with the final version released in 1998. There have been annual updates to the system since the final release.

The system underwent an informal test in October 1996, which was followed by a formal test conducted by HCFA to determine whether ICD-10-PCS would be a practical replacement for ICD-9-CM procedures. Clinical Data Abstraction Centers (CDACs) were trained on the use of

ICD-10-PCS and coded 5,000 records. They also compared ICD-9-CM and ICD-10-PCS codes. The CDACs found ICD-10-PCS to be an improvement over ICD-9-CM in that it provided greater specificity in coding for use in research, statistical analysis, and administrative areas. A major strength of the system is its detailed structure, which enables users to recognize and report more precisely the procedures that were performed.

Goals/Purpose

The purpose of ICD-10-PCS was to develop a superior procedure coding system to replace volume 3 of ICD-9-CM. The goal of ICD-10-PCS was to develop a system that incorporated four major attributes: completeness, expandability, multiaxial system, and standardized terminology. ICD-10-PCS has a multiaxial, seven-character, alphanumerical code structure, which provides a unique code for all substantially different procedures and allows new procedures to be easily incorporated as new codes.

Users of ICD-10-PCS

Even though the system is capable of classifying a multitude of procedure types, it is being implemented as the replacement for current volume 3 ICD-9-CM users. This means that hospital inpatient encounters will be coded with ICD-10-PCS procedure codes. Those currently using CPT/HCPCS codes (that is, physician offices, outpatient surgery, outpatient ancillary services, and such) will continue to use CPT/HCPCS codes. Note that ICD-10-PCS would not affect physicians, outpatient facilities, and hospital outpatient departments' usage of Current Procedural Terminology (CPT) codes on Medicare Fee for Service claims as CPT use would continue.

Essential Attributes

Development of ICD-10-PCS was based on four major objectives. These essential characteristics are shown in figure 3.1.

Figure 3.1. Essential characteristics of ICD-10-PCS

Characteristics	Explanation
Completeness	There should be a unique code for all substantially different procedures.
Expandability	As new procedures are developed, the structure of ICD-10-PCS should allow them to be easily incorporated as unique codes.
Multiaxial	The structure should be a multiaxial structure, with each individual axis having the same meaning within a specific procedure section and across procedure sections.
Standard Terminology	It should include definitions of the terminology used. Although the meaning of specific words can vary in common usage, ICD-10-PCS should not include multiple meanings for the same term and each term must be assigned a specific meaning.

Source: Development of the ICD-10 Procedure Coding System (ICD-10-PCS). 2009. http://www.cms.hhs.gov/ICD10/.

General Principles

Several general principles were followed in the development of the ICD-10-PCS system. They are:

- Diagnostic information is not included in procedure description
    - When procedures are performed for specific disorders or diseases, the disease or disorder is not contained in the procedure code.
- Not Otherwise Specified (NOS) options are restricted
    - Not Otherwise Specified (NOS) options are frequent in ICD-9-CM, but limited in ICD-10-PCS to those uses identified in the ICD-10-PCS Draft Guidelines. A minimal level of specificity is required for each component of the procedure.
- Limited use of Not Elsewhere Classified (NEC) option
    - Since all significant components of a procedure are specified in ICD-10-PCS, there is usually no need for an NEC code option. There is a limited NEC option incorporated into ICD-10-PCS where necessary. For example, new devices are frequently developed, and it may be necessary to use "Other Device" option until the new device is explicitly added to the system.
- Level of specificity
    - All procedures currently performed can be specified in ICD-10-PCS. The frequency with which a procedure is performed was

not a consideration in the development of the system. ICD-10-PCS has unique codes available for variations of a procedure that can be performed.

Source: Development of the ICD-10 Procedure Coding System (ICD-10-PCS). January 2009. Available on-line at www.cms.hhs.gov/ICD10/

Code Structure

ICD-10-PCS has a completely different structure than ICD-9-CM. Because ICD-10-PCS codes consist of individual values rather than lists of fixed codes and text descriptions, each code in the system has a unique definition. New values may be added to the system to represent a specific new approach, device, or qualifier, but whole codes are not reused and given new meanings. A brief comparison follows.

ICD-9-CM

ICD-9-CM has three to four numeric characters. A decimal is placed after the second character, and all codes must have at least three characters. For example:

43.5 – Partial gastrectomy with anastomosis to esophagus

44.42 – Suture of duodenal ulcer site

| 4 | 4 | . | 4 | 2 |

ICD-10-PCS

ICD-10-PCS has a seven-character alphanumeric code structure. Each character has many different possible values. The digits 0–9 and the letters *A–H, J–N*, and *P–Z* are used. The letters *O* and *I* are not used in order to avoid confusion with the digits 0 and 1. The letters and numbers are intermingled throughout the code, and any of the seven digits may be alpha or numeric. The alpha characters are not case sensitive. ICD-10-PCS does not utilize a decimal in its structure. It is important to note that each code in ICD-10-PCS MUST have seven characters. For example:

0FB03ZX – Excision of Liver, Percutaneous
            Approach, Diagnostic
0DQ10ZZ – Repair, upper esophagus

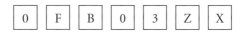

Procedures are divided into sections that relate to the general type of procedure (medical and surgical, imaging, obstetrics, nuclear medicine, and such). The first character of the procedure code always specifies the section.

The number of codes is extensive, with a total number estimated in the 2009 version at 72,589. There are approximately 4,000 ICD-9-CM procedure codes. This expansion of codes presents an opportunity to provide better data needed to meet the demands of an increasingly global and electronic healthcare environment. It also provides a significant opportunity to improve the capture of information about the increasingly complex delivery of healthcare. The increase in the numbers of codes does not make the system more difficult to use, in fact it is easier because there is an individual code available for each identified procedure. An analogy might be in using a dictionary. The size of a dictionary does not make it more difficult to use because you are referencing only a specific concept, not the entire publication. Having a complete, robust coding system actually makes it easier to find the correct code. The current coding process does not involve reviewing the entire list of ICD-9-CM codes in search of the proper code. The Alphabetic Index/Tables in ICD-10-PCS and electronic coding tools will continue to facilitate proper code selection. It is anticipated that the improved structure and specificity of ICD-10-PCS will facilitate the development of increasingly sophisticated electronic coding tools to aid in the process of code selection, resulting in less time spent on a manual code selection process than being used today. The greater specificity and clinical accuracy and a more logical structure actually make ICD-10-PCS easier to use than ICD-9-CM.

ICD-10-PCS Manual
The ICD-10-PCS online manual is divided into two main parts, the Index and the ICD-10-PCS Tables.

Figure 3.2. Grid example

0: MEDICAL AND SURGICAL
D: GASTROINTESTINAL SYSTEM
J: INSPECTION: Visually and/or manually exploring a body part

Body Part Character 4	Approach Character 5	Device Character 6	Qualifier Character 7
0 Upper intestinal Tract 1 Esophagus, Upper 2 Esophagus, Middle 3 Esophagus, Lower 4 Esophagogastric Junction 5 Esophagus 6 Stomach 7 Stomach, Pylorus 8 Small intestine 9 Duodenum A Jejunum B Ileum C Ileocecal Valve E Large Intestine F Large Intestine, Right G Large Intestine, Left H Cecum J Appendix K Ascending Colon L Transverse Colon M Descending Colon N Sigmoid Colon P Rectum Q Anus	0 Open 3 Percutaneous 4 Percutaneous Endoscopic 7 Via Natural or Artificial Opening 8 Via Natural or Artificial Opening Endoscopic X External	Z No Device	Z No Qualifier

0: MEDICAL AND SURGICAL D: GASTROINTESTINAL SYSTEM J: INSPECTION: Visually and/or manually exploring a body part			
Body Part Character 4	Approach Character 5	Device Character 6	Qualifier Character 7
R Anal Sphincter S Greater Omentum T Lesser Omentum V Mesentery W Peritoneum	0 Open 3 Percutaneous 4 Percutaneous Endoscopic X External	Z No Device	Z No Qualifier

System Structure

Procedures in ICD-10-PCS are divided into sections that relate to the general type of procedure. There are 16 sections in ICD-10-PCS. Each section identifies the general type of procedure; for example, medical and surgical. The first character of the procedure code always specifies the section or type of procedure. The second through seventh characters have a standard meaning within each section but may have a different meaning across sections. In ICD-10-PCS, the term *procedure* is used to refer to the complete specification of the seven characters. All terminology in ICD-10-PCS is defined precisely, with a specific meaning attached to all terms used in the system. See figure 3.3.

Figure 3.3. Sections of ICD-10-PCS

Section	Title
0	Medical and Surgical
1	Obstetrics
2	Placement
3	Administration
4	Measurement and Monitoring
5	Extracorporeal Assistance and Performance
6	Extracorporeal Therapies
7	Osteopathic
8	Other Procedures
9	Chiropractic
B	Imaging
C	Nuclear Medicine
D	Radiation Oncology
F	Physical Rehabilitation and Diagnostic Audiology
G	Mental Health
H	Substance Abuse Treatment

Source: Centers for Medicare & Medicaid Services. 2009. ICD-10-PCS. http://www.cms.hhs.gov/ICD10.

Code Characters in the Medical and Surgical Section

The medical and surgical procedures section contains most, but not all, procedures typically reported in the hospital inpatient setting, and the following figure demonstrates the meanings of the seven characters in this section. However, it is important to remember that the characters have a slightly different meaning in each section, but that they are well defined in the coding system.

Meaning of Characters for Medical and Surgical Procedures

1	2	3	4	5	6	7

Section — Body System — Root Operation — Body Part — Approach — Device — Qualifier

Section

In the medical and surgical procedures section, the first character of the code specifying the section is 0.

Body System

The second character defines the body system, the general physiological system, or anatomical region involved. The endocrine system is an example of a body system. This way of categorizing into larger groupings makes the tables easier to navigate and provides information quickly about the procedure. All procedures with the same second character would be of the same anatomical region or system, facilitating data comparisons.

Some traditional categories are subdivided into several body systems. (See figure 3.4.) For example, the cardiovascular system is subdivided into five systems:

- Heart and great vessels
- Upper arteries
- Lower arteries
- Upper veins
- Lower veins

Figure 3.4. ICD-10-PCS medical and surgical section (0) body systems

Character	Title
0	Central Nervous Systems
1	Peripheral Nervous Systems
2	Heart and Great Vessels
3	Upper Arteries
4	Lower Arteries
5	Upper Veins
6	Lower Veins
7	Lymphatic and Hemic System
8	Eye
9	Ear, Nose, Sinus
B	Respiratory System
C	Mouth and Throat
D	Gastrointestinal System
F	Hepatobiliary System and Pancreas
G	Endocrine System
H	Skin and Breast
J	Subcutaneous Tissue and fascia
K	Muscles
L	Tendons
M	Bursae and ligaments
N	Head and Facial Bones
P	Upper Bones
Q	Lower Bones
R	Upper Joints
S	Lower Joints
T	Urinary System
U	Female Reproductive System

Character	Title
V	Male Reproductive System
W	Anatomical Regions, General
X	Anatomical Regions, Upper Extremities
Y	Anatomical Regions, Lower Extremities

Source: Centers for Medicare & Medicaid Services. 2009. ICD-10-PCS. http://www.cms.hhs.gov/ICD10.

Root Operation

The third character indicates the root operation, which specifies the objective of the procedure (for example, excision). ICD-10-PCS has done an exemplary job of defining these terms. It also has included examples of each term for clarification. There currently are 31 root operations, and they are arranged by groups with similar attributes. If multiple procedures as defined by distinct objectives are performed, then multiple codes are assigned.

A root operation must specify the objective of the procedure. The term *anastomosis* is not a root operation because it is a means of joining and is an integral part of another procedure such as a bypass or a resection; therefore, it can never stand alone. Incision is not a root term because it is a means of opening and is always an integral part of another procedure. Repair is only coded when none of the other operations apply and is therefore the NEC option for the root operation character. It is used when documentation and necessary information cannot be obtained from the physician indicating a more specific root operation. See figure 3.5.

Figure 3.5. Root operations with definitions

Operation		Definition, Explanation, Examples
Alteration 0	Definition	Modifying the natural anatomic structure of a body part without affecting the function of the body part
	Explanation	Principal purpose is to improve appearance
	Examples	Face-lift, breast augmentation
Bypass 1	Definition	Altering the route of passage of the contents of a tubular body part
	Explanation	Rerouting contents around an area of a body part to another distal (downstream) area in the normal route; rerouting the contents to another different, but similar, route and body part or to an abnormal route and another dissimilar body part. It includes one or more concurrent anastomoses with or without the use of devices such as autografts, tissue substitutes, and synthetic substitutes.
	Examples	Coronary artery bypass, colostomy formation

Operation		Definition, Explanation, Examples
Change 2	Definition	Taking out or off a device from a body part and putting back an identical or similar device in or on the same body part without cutting or puncturing the skin or a mucous membrane
	Explanation	All change procedures are coded using the approach External
	Examples	Urinary catheter change, gastrostomy tube change
Control 3	Definition	Stopping, or attempting to stop, postprocedural bleeding
	Explanation	The site of the bleeding is coded as an anatomical region and not to a specific body part.
	Examples	Control of postprostatectomy hemorrhage, control of post-tonsillectomy hemorrhage
Creation 4	Definition	Making a new genital structure that does not physically take the place of a body part
	Explanation	Used only for sex change operations
	Examples	Creation of vagina in a male, creation of penis in a female

Operation		Definition, Explanation, Examples
Destruction 5	Definition	Physical eradication of all or a portion of a body part by the direct use of energy, force, or a destructive agent
	Explanation	None of the body part is physically taken out.
	Examples	Fulguration of rectal polyp, cautery of skin lesion
Detachment 6	Definition	Cutting off all or a portion of the upper or lower extremities
	Explanation	The body part value is the site of the detachment, with a qualifier if applicable to further specify the level where the extremity was detached.
	Examples	Below-knee amputation, disarticulation of shoulder
Dilation 7	Definition	Expanding an orifice or the lumen of a tubular body part
	Explanation	The orifice can be a natural orifice or an artificially created orifice. Accomplished by stretching a tubular body part using intraluminal pressure or by cutting part of the orifice or wall of the tubular body part.
	Examples	Percutaneous transluminal angioplasty, pyloromyotomy

Operation		Definition, Explanation, Examples
Division 8	Definition	Cutting into a body part without draining fluids and/or gases from the body part in order to separate or transect a body part.
	Explanation	All or a portion of the body part is separated into two or more portions.
	Examples	Spinal cordotomy, osteotomy
Drainage 9	Definition	Taking or letting out fluids and/or gases from a body part
	Explanation	The qualifier Diagnostic is used to identify drainage procedures that are biopsies.
	Examples	Thoracentesis, incision and drainage
Excision B	Definition	Cutting out or off, without replacement, a portion of a body part
	Explanation	The qualifier Diagnostic is used to identify excision procedures that are biopsies.
	Examples	Partial nephrectomy, liver biopsy

Operation		Definition, Explanation, Examples
Extirpation C	Definition	Taking or cutting out solid matter from a body part
	Explanation	The solid matter may be an abnormal byproduct of a biological function or a foreign body. The solid matter is imbedded in a body part or is in the lumen of a tubular body part. The solid matter may or may not have been previously broken into pieces. No appreciable amount of the body part is taken out.
	Examples	Thrombectomy, choledocho-lithotomy
Extraction D	Definition	Pulling or stripping out or off all or a portion of a body part by the use of force
	Explanation	The qualifier Diagnostic is used to identify extractions that are biopsies.
	Examples	Dilation and curettage, vein stripping

Operation		Definition, Explanation, Examples
Fragmentation F	Definition	Breaking solid matter in a body part into pieces
	Explanation	The solid matter may be an abnormal byproduct of a biological function or a foreign body. Physical force (for example, manual, ultrasonic) applied directly or indirectly through intervening body parts is used to break the solid matter into pieces. The pieces of solid matter are not taken out, but are eliminated or absorbed through normal biological functions.
	Examples	Extracorporeal shockwave lithotripsy, transurethral lithotripsy
Fusion G	Definition	Joining together portions of an articular body part rendering the articular body part immobile
	Explanation	The body part is joined together by fixation device, bone graft, or other means
	Examples	Spinal fusion, ankle arthrodesis
Insertion H	Definition	Putting in a nonbiological appliance that monitors, assists, performs, or prevents a physiological function but does not physically take the place of a body part
	Explanation	N/A
	Examples	Insertion of radioactive implant, insertion of central venous catheter

Operation		Definition, Explanation, Examples
Inspection J	Definition	Visually and/or manually exploring a body part
	Explanation	Visual exploration may be performed with or without optical instrumentation. Manual exploration may be performed directly or through intervening body layers.
	Examples	Diagnostic arthroscopy, exploratory laparotomy
Map K	Definition	Locating the route of passage of electrical impulses and/or locating functional areas in a body part
	Explanation	Applicable only to the cardiac conduction mechanism and the central nervous system
	Examples	Cardiac mapping, cortical mapping
Occlusion L	Definition	Completely closing an orifice or the lumen of a tubular body part
	Explanation	The orifice can be a natural orifice or an artificially created orifice
	Examples	Fallopian tube ligation, ligation of inferior vena cava

Operation		Definition, Explanation, Examples
Reattachment M	Definition	Putting back in or on all or a portion of a separated body part to its normal location or other suitable location
	Explanation	Vascular circulation and nervous pathways may or may not be reestablished.
	Examples	Reattachment of hand, reattachment of avulsed kidney
Release N	Definition	Freeing a body part from an abnormal physical constraint by cutting or by use of force
	Explanation	Some of the restraining tissue may be taken out, but none of the body part is taken out.
	Examples	Adhesiolysis, carpal tunnel release
Removal P	Definition	Taking out or off a device from a body part
	Explanation	If the device is taken out and a similar device is put in without cutting or puncturing the skin or mucous membrane, the procedure is coded to the root operation CHANGE. Otherwise, the procedure for taking out the device is coded to the root operation REMOVAL, and the procedure for putting in the new device is coded to the root operation performed.
	Examples	Drainage tube removal, cardiac pacemaker removal

Operation		Definition, Explanation, Examples
Repair Q	Definition	Restoring, to the extent possible, a body part to its normal anatomic structure and function
	Explanation	Used only when the method to accomplish the repair is not one of the other root operations
	Examples	Herniorrhaphy, suture of laceration
Replacement R	Definition	Putting in or on biological or synthetic material that physically takes the place and/or function of all or a portion of a body part
	Explanation	The biological material is nonliving or the biological material is living and from the same individual. The body part may have been previously taken out, previously replaced, or may be taken out concomitantly with the replacement procedure. If the body part has been previously replaced, a separate removal procedure is coded for taking out the device used in the previous replacement.
	Examples	Total hip replacement, bone graft, free skin graft

Operation		Definition, Explanation, Examples
Reposition S	Definition	Moving to its normal location or other suitable location all or a portion of a body part
	Explanation	The body part is moved to a new location from an abnormal location, or from a normal location where it is not functioning correctly. The body part may or may not be cut out or off to be moved to the new location.
	Examples	Reposition of undescended testicle, fracture reduction
Resection T	Definition	Cutting out or off, without replacement, all of a body part
	Explanation	N/A
	Examples	Total nephrectomy, total lobectomy of lung
Restriction V	Definition	Partially closing an orifice or the lumen of a tubular body part
	Explanation	The orifice can be a natural orifice or an artificially created orifice.
	Examples	Esophagogastric fundoplication, cervical cerclage

Operation		Definition, Explanation, Examples
Revision W	Definition	Correcting, to the extent possible, a malfunctioning or displaced device
	Explanation	Revision can include correcting a malfunctioning or displaced device by taking out or putting in components of the device such as a screw or pin
	Examples	Adjustment of pacemaker lead, adjustment of hip prosthesis
Supplement U	Definition	Putting in or on biologic or synthetic material that physically reinforces and/or augments the function of a portion of a body part
	Explanation	The biological material is nonliving, or the biological material is living and from the same individual. The body part may have been previously replaced. If the body part has been previously replaced, the supplement procedure is performed to physically reinforce and/or augment the function of the replaced body part.
	Examples	Herniorrhaphy using mesh, free nerve graft, mitral valve ring annuloplasty, put a new acetabular liner in a previous hip replacement

Operation		Definition, Explanation, Examples
Transfer X	Definition	Moving, without taking out, all or a portion of a body part to another location to take over the function of all or a portion of a body part
	Explanation	The body part transferred remains connected to its vascular and nervous supply.
	Examples	Tendon transfer, skin pedicle flap transfer
Transplantation Y	Definition	Putting in or on all or a portion of a living body part taken from another individual or animal to physically take the place and/or function of all or a portion of a similar body part
	Explanation	The native body part may or may not be taken out, and the transplanted body part may take over all or a portion of its function.
	Examples	Kidney transplant, heart transplant

Source: Centers for Medicare & Medicaid Services. 2009.
Development of the ICD-10 Procedure Coding System
(ICD-10-PCS). http://www.cms.hhs.gov/ICD10.

Body Part

The body part is specified in the fourth character and indicates the specific part of the body system on which the procedure was performed (for example, stomach). This is the specific site, different from character 2, which provided the general body system. There are 34 possible body part values in each body system.

Examples of body parts:
- Liver
- Kidney
- Thalamus
- Ascending Colon
- Optic Nerve
- Tonsil

Approach

The fifth character indicates the approach or the technique of the procedure. There are seven different approach values in the medical and surgical section.

Approaches may be through the skin or mucous membrane, through an orifice, or external. See figure 3.6.

Figure 3.6. Surgical approaches

Approach Description Value	Approach Definition
Open (0)	Cutting through the skin or mucous membrane and any other body layers necessary to expose the site of the procedure
Percutaneous (3)	Entry, by puncture or minor incision, of instrumentation through the skin or mucous membrane and any other body layers necessary to reach the site of the procedure
Percutaneous Endoscopic (4)	Entry, by puncture or minor incision, of instrumentation through the skin or mucous membrane and any other body layers necessary to reach and visualize the site of the procedure
Via Natural or Artificial Opening (7)	Entry of instrumentation through a natural or artificial external opening to reach the site of the procedure
Via Natural or Artificial Opening Endoscopic (8)	Entry of instrumentation through a natural or artificial external opening to reach and visualize the site of the procedure
Via Natural or Artificial Opening with Percutaneous Endoscopic Assistance (F)	Entry of instrumentation through a natural or artificial external opening and entry, by puncture or minor incision, of instrumentation through the skin or mucous membrane and any other body layers necessary to aid in the performance of the procedure
External (X)	Procedures performed directly on the skin or mucous membrane and procedures performed indirectly by the application of external force through the skin or mucous membrane

Source: Centers for Medicare & Medicaid Services.
ICD-10 Procedure Coding System (ICD-10-PCS). 2009.
http://www.cms.hhs.gov/ICD10.

Device

The device is specified in the sixth character and is only used to specify devices that remain after the procedure is completed. If no device is applicable, the letter *Z* is used.

Device values fall into four basic groups:
1. Grafts and Prostheses
2. Implants
3. Simple or Mechanical Appliances
4. Electronic Appliances

There are four general types of devices:
1. Biological or synthetic material that takes the place of all or a portion of a body part (skin grafts and joint prosthesis)
2. Biological or synthetic material that assists or prevents a physiological function (IUD)
3. Therapeutic material that is not absorbed by, eliminated by, or incorporated into a body part (radioactive implant)
4. Mechanical or electronic appliances used to assist, monitor, take the place of, or prevent a physiological function (cardiac pacemaker, orthopedic pins)

Qualifier

The seventh character is for the qualifier. The qualifier has a unique meaning for individual procedures. It could be used to identify the second site included in a bypass or to identify that a biopsy is a diagnostic procedure. These qualifiers may have a narrow application, to a specific root operation, body system, or body part. Most procedures will not have an applicable qualifier. The default value to indicate that NO qualifier is needed is Z.

Examples of Qualifiers
- Type of transplant
- Second site for a bypass
- Diagnostic excision (biopsy)

Medical and Surgical Code Examples

The table below provides examples of codes from the medical and surgical section. Any specific clinical knowledge required is noted in the comments column. The character values for each of these codes can be obtained by accessing the ICD-10-PCS system on the CMS Web site. See figure 3.7.

Figure 3.7. Medical and surgical code examples

Procedure	ICD-10-PCS Code	Comments
Percutaneous transluminal coronary angioplasty of two coronary arteries: left anterior descending artery with stent placement and right coronary artery with no stent	02703DZ 02703ZZ	A separate procedure is coded for each artery dilated, since the device value differs for each artery.
Open posterior tarsal tunnel release	01NG0ZZ	Nerve released in posterior tarsal tunnel is the tibial nerve.
Sigmoidoscopy with sigmoid polypectomy	0DBN8ZZ	
Fifth ray carpometacarpal joint amputation, left hand	0X6K0Z8	Qualifier value for complete fifth ray is used because a complete ray amputation is through the carpometacarpal joint.
Percutaneous placement of Swan-Ganz catheter in superior vena cava	02HV32Z	Swan-Ganz catheter is coded to the device value "monitoring device" because it monitors pulmonary artery output.
Placement of intrathecal infusion pump for pain management, percutaneous	0JHT33Z	This device resides principally in the subcutaneous tissue of the back, so it is coded to the subcutaneous and fascia body system.

Procedure	ICD-10-PCS Code	Comments
Endoscopic retrograde cholangiopancreatography (ERCP) with lithotripsy of common bile duct stone	0FF98ZZ	ERCP is performed through the mouth to the biliary system via the duodenum, so the approach value is via natural or artificial opening, endoscopic.
Right shoulder arthroscopy with coracoacromial ligament release	0MN14ZZ	The body part value for right coracoacromial ligament is shoulder bursa and ligament, right.
Fasciocutaneous flap closure of left thigh, open	0JXM0ZC	The qualifier identifies the body layers that are included in the procedure (skin, subcutaneous tissue, and fascia).
Percutaneous biopsy of right gastrocnemius muscle	0KBS3ZX	The body part value is lower leg muscle, right. The root operation is excision, and the qualifier indicates diagnostic to denote that this is a biopsy.
Endoscopic left leg flexor hallucis longus tendon transfer	0LXP4ZZ	The body part value is lower leg tendon, left.

Procedure	ICD-10-PCS Code	Comments
Uterine artery embolization	04LE3DZ	Since the uterine artery is not identified by a separate body part value, it is coded to the closest proximal branch identified by a body part value (the left internal iliac artery).
Suture repair of right biceps tendon laceration, open	0LQ30ZZ	The body part value is upper arm tendon, right.
Carpal tunnel release, percutaneous endoscopic	01N54ZZ	The body part value is median nerve.

Comparison Between ICD-9-CM and ICD-10-PCS Procedures

As previously discussed, ICD-10-PCS is an entirely new system, and as such, the codes do not have a similar structure or appearance. Mapping between the systems is not an easy process, discussed in more detail in chapter 5.

The increased detail available in the ICD-10-PCS codes has been discussed previously in this chapter, but it may be helpful to review a few ICD-9-CM codes with their counterpart ICD-10-PCS codes to identify the additional detail available in the new coding system (such as with approach and specificity). See figure 3.8.

Figure 3.8. Comparison between ICD-9-CM and ICD-10-PCS procedures

Procedure	ICD-9-CM Code	ICD-10-PCS Code	Comments/ Comparisons
Suture right internal carotid artery, open	39.31 Suture of artery No other detail or choices available	03QK0ZZ 0 = Med/Surg 3 = Upper arteries Q = Repair K = Right internal carotid artery 0 = Open approach Z = No device Z = No qualifier	The ICD-9-CM code 39.31 does not identify the specific artery sutured or the approach. All repairs classify to the same code. Any sutures of arteries code to 39.31. The ICD-10-PCS code identifies each individual artery and specifies laterality, and approach used (open, percutaneous, percutaneous endoscopic). There are 65 different arteries identified in PCS and 195 different specific codes possible for ICD-9-CM code 39.31.

Procedure	ICD-9-CM Code	ICD-10-PCS Code	Comments/ Comparisons
Excisional debridement of left heel skin ulcer	86.22 Excisional debridement of wound, infection, or burn No other detail or choices available	0HBNXZZ 0 = Med/Surg H = Skin & Breast B = Excision N = Skin, Left Foot X = External Z = No device Z = No qualifier	The ICD-9-CM code 86.22 does not identify any specific site of the skin. There are 31 specific sites that can be identified, including the laterality.
Open reduction, internal fixation displaced left tarsal fracture	79.37 Open reduction of fracture with internal fixation tarsals and metatarsals	0QSM04Z 0 = Med/Surg Q = Lower Bones S = Reposition M = Tarsal, Left 0 = Open 4 = Internal Fixation Device Z = No device	The ICD-9-CM code does provide information on approach (open) or that internal fixation was done. The fourth digit however includes tarsals and metatarsals, so it does not specify which one, and it does not provide laterality. ICD-10-PCS provides specific values for tarsal and metatarsals, as well as the laterality of each.

Procedure	ICD-9-CM Code	ICD-10-PCS Code	Comments/ Comparisons
Open excision of retained metal, subcutaneous tissue right hand	86.05 Incision with removal of foreign body or device from skin and subcutaneous tissue No other detail or choices available	0JCJ0ZZ 0 = Med/Surg J = Subcutaneous Tissue and Fascia C = Extirpation J = Right Hand 0 = Open Z = No Device Z = No Qualifier	The ICD-9-CM code includes removal of foreign bodies of either the skin or the subcutaneous tissue without differentiation or without the specific site identified. In ICD-10-PCS there are different codes for specific body systems for skin and subcutaneous tissues, as well as specific part sites in each, including laterality. In addition, removal of a device has a special root operation, while removal of foreign body classifies to the root operation extirpation.

Procedure	ICD-9-CM Code	ICD-10-PCS Code	Comments/ Comparisons
PTCA of three coronary arteries using drug eluting stents	00.66 PTCA or coronary atherectomy 00.42 Procedure on three vessels 00.47 Insertion of three vascular stents 36.07 Insertion of drug-eluting coronary artery stents(s)	027234Z 0 = Med/Surg 2 = Heart and Great Vessels 7 = Dilation 2 = Coronary Artery, Three sites 3 = Percutaneous 4 = Drug-eluting Intraluminal Device Z = No Qualifier	In this example, it requires four different codes in ICD-9-CM to classify the same procedure reported with one ICD-10-PCS code

Procedures Outside Medical and Surgical Section

Most procedures typically reported in an inpatient setting can be found in the medical and surgical section of ICD-10-PCS. However, a number of significant procedures that are currently reported with ICD-9-CM procedure codes can be found in other sections. As with medical and surgical codes, the character values for each of these codes can be obtained by accessing the ICD-10-PCS system on the Centers for Medicare and Medicaid Services Web site.

There are two primary additional sections in ICD-10-PCS, the medical and surgical-related sections of ICD-10-PCS and procedures in the ancillary sections. The compositions are listed below in figures 3.9 and 3.10, and a code examples are shown in figure 3.11.

Figure 3.9. Medical and surgical-related sections of ICD-10-PCS

Section Value	Description
1	Obstetrics
2	Placement
3	Administration
4	Measurement and Monitoring
5	Extracorporeal Assistance and Performance
6	Extracorporeal Therapies
7	Osteopathic
8	Other Procedures
9	Chiropractic

Figure 3.10. Procedures in the ancillary sections

Section Value	Description
B	Imaging
C	Nuclear Medicine
D	Radiation Oncology
F	Physical Rehabilitation and Diagnostic Audiology
G	Mental Health
H	Substance Abuse Treatment

Figure 3.11. Medical and surgical-related section code examples

Procedure	ICD-10-PCS Code	Comments
Bone marrow transplant using donor marrow from sibling, central venous infusion	30243G1	The "3" in the first character position indicates the administration section. Character "6" in the administration section identifies substance (for example, bone marrow).
Esophagogastroscopy with Botox injection into esophageal sphincter	3E0G8GC	Botulinum toxin is a paralyzing agent with temporary effects; it does not sclerose or destroy the nerve.
Epidural injection of mixed steroid and local anesthetic for pain control	3E0S33Z	The substance value anti-inflammatory is used because the anesthetic is only added to lessen the pain of the injection.

Procedure	ICD-10-PCS Code	Comments
Pulsatile compression boot with intermittent inflation	5A02115	The "5" in the first character position indicates the extracorporeal assistance and performance section. The root operation "0" is assistance (taking over a portion of a physiological function by extracorporeal means). The function value (character 6) is coded to cardiac output because the purpose of such compression devices is to return blood to the heart faster.

Procedure	ICD-10-PCS Code	Comments
Open in utero repair of congenital diaphragmatic hernia	10Q00ZK	The "1" in the first character position indicates the obstetrics section. In ICD-10-PCS, the diaphragm is considered part of the respiratory system, so the qualifier (the seventh character) indicates that the procedure was performed on the respiratory system (the body part value indicates that the procedure was performed on the fetus).
Intermittent mechanical ventilation, 20 hours	5A0935Z	

ICD-10-PCS Guidelines

ICD-10-PCS draft coding guidelines were developed for ICD-10-PCS and are available at http://www.cms.hhs.gov/ICD10/. They are grouped into general guidelines and guidelines that apply to a section or sections. Guidelines for the Medical and Surgical section are further grouped by character. The guidelines are numbered sequentially within each category.

Additional Clinical Knowledge Required

In many cases, more extensive knowledge of anatomy and physiology, the clinical performance of a procedure, and the purpose of devices is needed for ICD-10-PCS code assignment than is required for ICD-9-CM coding.

Complete documentation of a procedure will also be important to accurately assign the code. ICD-10-PCS appears to provide more complete and accurate descriptions of the procedures performed than volume 3 of ICD-9-CM. All procedures on a particular body part, by a particular approach, or by another characteristic can be easily retrieved using ICD-10-PCS data. The codes will provide very specific information about a particular procedure.

Body part values for muscles and tendons are defined by anatomical site (for example, upper leg muscle, upper leg tendon) instead of name. If the procedure report identifies the muscle or tendon by the Latin anatomical name (for example, soleus muscle), an understanding of anatomy and access to an anatomy reference will be needed to select the appropriate body part value. According to the ICD-10-PCS draft coding guidelines, nerves and vessels that are not identified by a separate body part value are coded to the closest proximal branch identified by a body part value. This may require anatomy review and ongoing access to an anatomy reference. For example, the superior laryngeal nerve is a branch of the vagus nerve, so a procedure performed on the superior laryngeal nerve is coded to the body part value for vagus nerve. Detailed knowledge of anatomy is also needed to assign the appropriate body part value for bones and joints.

Chapter 4
Impact of the Transition

The benefits of ICD-10-CM and ICD-10-PCS and the necessity of the transition to the new code sets has previously been discussed in this guide, however the implementation will present a number of challenges. Adoption of ICD-10-CM/PCS as the national code set presents numerous issues in terms of budgeting and managing the implementation, training personnel to use the code sets and adapting current information systems to accept the different formats.

Although the implementation date for ICD-10-CM/PCS is not until 2013, it is not too early to begin planning for the transition, and even putting some of those plans in motion. A well-planned, well-managed implementation process will increase the chances of a smooth, successful transition. Experience in other countries has shown that early preparation is key to success. The best way to manage the challenges inherent in making a transition of this magnitude is to engage in them in a phased approach.

Some of the preparation activities necessary for implementation provide benefits to the organization even before ICD-10-CM/PCS are implemented, such as medical record documentation improvement strategies and efforts to expand coding staff knowledge and skills. Also, an early start allows for resource allocation, such as costs for systems changes and education as well as staff time devoted to implementation processes, to be spread over several years. Thus, many of the costs can be absorbed by existing annual budgets rather than requiring a large budgetary investment at one time.

Preparing for ICD-10-CM/PCS

A thorough implementation plan that is established and begun well in advance of the scheduled implementation date is necessary to ensure a successful transition to ICD-10-CM/PCS. For more information on steps to prepare for implementation, review AHIMA's ICD-10 Preparation Checklist (http://www.ahima. org/ICD10/ICD-10preparationchecklist.mht) also available in Appendix A of this guide.

Since many countries have already implemented ICD-10, it may be helpful to review lessons learned during their transition. Keep in mind that the United States is the only country using ICD-10-CM/PCS, so comparisons are not entirely reliable. For more information, including accounts of Canada and Australia's implementations, review the following AHIMA articles (available at www. ahima.org/icd10/links.html under Collection of Articles in the Body of Knowledge on ICD-10).

- What's your ICD-10 Plan? Findings and Recommendations from Research on ICD-10 (February 2005)
- Planning and Implementing ICD-10, Using a Team Approach (October 2004)

- The Implementation of ICD-10-CA and CCI in Canada (October 2004)
- A Time for Change—A Time for Ten: Updating the Classification for Discharges On and After 1.1.05 to ICD-10-AM (October 2004)
- ICD-10: An Update on the Worldwide Implementation—the Australian Experience (October 2004)
- Destination 10: Healthcare Organization Preparation for ICD-10-CM and ICD-10-PCS (March 2004)
- Ten Down Under: Implementing ICD-10 in Australia (January 2000)

Who Will Be Affected by the Implementation of ICD-10-CM/PCS

All users of ICD-9-CM data will be impacted by this transition, but to varying degrees depending on the extent of their involvement. Certainly, the knowledge required will be dependent on current uses of the systems. For example, an inpatient coding professional will require in-depth training on how to code with both new systems, while clinicians will need education on new documentation requirements. Also, different categories of coding professionals will require varying levels of training. ICD-10-CM will be used in all settings, so all coding professionals will require training on this system, while only hospital inpatient coders will require intensive training on ICD-10-PCS.

The following is a list of data users requiring some level of education. Note that this list is not all-inclusive, but can be customized within each organization.

- Coding Professionals
- All HIM staff
- Physicians
- Clinicians other than physicians, such as nurses and allied health professionals
- Senior management
- Information systems
- Quality management
- Case management
- Utilization management
- Accounting
- Business Services
- Patient access and registration
- Clinical department managers
- Ancillary departments
- Data analysts
- Performance improvement
- Compliance
- Data quality management
- Data security
- Data analysts
- Internal and external auditors and consultants
- Researchers
- Epidemiologists
- Software vendors
- Payers and insurance
- Fraud investigators
- Government agency personnel including Recovery Audit Contractors (RACs)

Certainly, all healthcare professionals who provide patient care should receive some level of training in ICD-10-CM and in ICD-10-PCS if applicable.

Students enrolled in HIM programs will need to be trained in both the ICD-9-CM and ICD-10-CM/PCS classification systems even after ICD-10-CM/PCS has been implemented so that they will be able to manage ICD-9-CM-based historical data.

In order to prepare these future students, educators in coding certificate, health information technology, and health information administration programs will be charged with the task of training new coding professionals.

The implementation of ICD-10-CM will benefit researchers and data analysts because ICD-10-CM will require concise and specific documentation from physicians and other clinical practitioners. In addition, because of its specificity with an individual code for each procedure and added detail, ICD-10-PCS will aid researchers and data analysts. Better data will improve the ability of providers, payers, the government, and others to measure the quality, safety, and efficiency of care; support providers' and payers' performance improvement activities; improve public health surveillance; and enhance health policy decision making. Some data analysts are already using ICD-10. For example, data analysts who work with international data are familiar with the system.

How Data Users Are Impacted

Many processes will be impacted because of the difference in the classification systems and changes in definitions and structure. Some of the key implementation issues to be considered are:

- Training of coding professionals and all other users
- Policy/procedure revisions
- Changes to multiple information systems and applications
- Increase in system storage capacity
- Redesign of reports and forms
- Modification of patient assessment data sets
- Impact on productivity and accuracy
- Data trending challenges

During planning for implementation, it will be important to complete an impact assessment of all data users and identify their specific use case to provide the specific education needed. The impact will be different depending on the specific use identified. Some examples of education requirements include:

- Senior management on requirements for standard code sets, with particular attention paid to implementation dates; HIPAA legislation; outline of impact to the organization; overview of differences between code sets; identification of time, effort, and resources required to implement changes; potential costs for implementation

- Clinicians on documentation requirements and changes to system, particularly new codes available in the system to classify conditions previously unreported
- Data security personnel on awareness of new codes to interpret software codes used to flag records
- Quality management, utilization review on differences in systems that impact work such as documentation requirements, longitudinal reporting, and time frames involved in changeover
- Other HIM staff on any codes that might impact their work such as sensitive information codes for release of information processes
- Vendors to ensure they are keeping up with the changes and obtain written contract (current and new) that updates and changes will be provided at no additional cost or limited cost; identify impacts to any new systems purchased

In addition to the impact on users of data, many current processes will be impacted. Consider the following processes in the implementation planning:

- Conversion of payment methodologies dependent on diagnosis/procedure codes
- National and local coverage determinations and code changes identified
- System logic and edits (that is, medical necessity)
- Provider profiling

- Quality measurement
- Utilization management
- Disease management
- Fraud management
- Aggregate data reporting

Training for Coding Professionals

Although ICD-10-CM is different from ICD-9-CM in many ways, the new classification system retains the traditional format and many of the same characteristics and conventions. Thus, experienced coding professionals should have little difficulty in achieving coding proficiency. Experienced coding professionals will require education on changes in the structure of the codes, disease classifications, definitions, and guidelines. For coders requiring training on the ICD-10-PCS system (hospital inpatient coding professionals), remember that ICD-10-PCS is entirely new, and will require intense training for proficiency. Additional education on anatomy and physiology, medical terminology, pharmacology, and medical science is needed.

There are many more trained coding professionals today than there were when ICD-9-CM was introduced, but less experienced users will face a number of challenges. The increased level of specificity with ICD-10-CM/PCS will require a strong foundation in anatomy and physiology, medical terminology, pharmacology, and medical science. The lead time before the implementation date of October 1, 2013 can be utilized to increase this knowledge.

Multiple categories of users of coded data and different categories of coders will require varying levels of training. Coding professionals working in settings that will not be using ICD-10-PCS will only require ICD-10-CM training, and that training may even be more specialized since physician practice coders working in a medical specialty area can be focused on particular code categories related to their practice.

For the intense training for experienced coders on how to actually code in the systems, it is suggested that this occur six to nine months prior to implementation in order to retain the information. There are several different projections regarding training needs, but according to the "HIPAA Administrative Simplifications: Modifications to Medical Data Code Set Standards To Adopt ICD-10-CM and ICD-10-PCS" Final Rule, training for experienced inpatient coders is estimated at 50 hours. CMS also calculated that experienced outpatient coders would need eight to ten hours of training time. These recommended hours of training presumes that coding professionals already possess the required knowledge in the biomedical sciences that will be needed to correctly apply codes using the ICD-10-CM/PCS systems.

An additional problem that could be encountered is a shortage of credentialed coding professionals. Currently, there is a shortage of coding professionals skilled in both ICD-9-CM and CPT® coding, but the implementation of ICD-10-CM/PCS offers significant job opportunities for students and professionals alike.

Training for Physicians

The inadequacy of physician documentation has been an obstacle for complete and accurate coding for some time. With the increased specificity in ICD-10-CM/PCS, complete documentation will be a factor in the collection of accurate statistical data as well as the key to appropriate reimbursement. A careful review of the code changes for ICD-10-CM/PCS clearly demonstrates the necessity of complete documentation and the use of current terminology. Having physicians actively involved in the implementation process allows them the opportunity to understand the importance of complete and accurate health record documentation.

While it is possible to assign nonspecific codes in the new systems, utilizing the full capabilities of these code sets will allow increased detail to enable more accurate and specific data. More detailed documentation will result in a more accurate clinical picture and better data for supporting the many purposes for which coded data are used today and will be used in the future such as:

- Measuring quality, safety and efficacy of care
- Designing payment systems and processing claims for reimbursement
- Conducting research, epidemiological studies, and clinical trials
- Setting health policy
- Operational and strategic planning and designing healthcare delivery systems
- Monitoring resource utilization

- Improving clinical, financial, and administrative performance
- Preventing and detecting healthcare fraud and abuse
- Tracking public health and risks
- Allowing increased computerization such as computer-assisted coding technologies

In addition to the training methods previously discussed, documentation assessment will continue to be an important tool for improving physician documentation. Results of the assessments can be shared with the physicians, and instances where patient care was compromised or revenue was lost because of inadequate documentation can be highlighted. Information on the uses of coded data apart from reimbursement should be shared with physicians as well so that they can better understand the impact of documentation.

ICD-10-CM/PCS Implementation Planning

The ICD-10 Preparation Checklist in Appendix A provides a systematic, detailed guide to managing the transition project through four stages of implementation, with specific strategies for each phase. A brief synopsis is provided here. The phases are:

- Phase 1 – Impact Assessment
- Phase 2 – Overall Implementation
- Phase 3 – Go-Live Preparation
- Phase 4 – Post-implementation

During the implementation planning there are seven key actions.

1. Develop strategy – establish a planning team, project leader, and physician champion and develop internal timelines and implementation plans

2. Communicate – build awareness and develop ongoing communication channels regarding the implementation plan and its progress (that is, newsletter, intranet)

3. Assess readiness – of affected staff, information systems and documentation process and workflow

4. Inventory process/system impact – identify all processes and systems impacted by the transition

5. Plan training – address education needs regarding type and level of education required, and how the education will be delivered

6. Documentation improvement – identify medical record documentation improvement opportunities and analyze ICD-9-CM frequency data and focus education efforts on most frequently-coded conditions

7. Develop budget – identify departmental budget responsibilities for costs of systems, hardware, software, and education. Analyze any increased staffing needs related to productivity and accuracy, either short-term or long-term and costs. Identify if consulting services will be needed for backlogs, monitoring coding accuracy or other support, and allocate this over a several year timeframe.

For more information on ICD-10-CM/PCS transition, review the article "Planning Organizational Transition to ICD-10-CM/PCS" in the October 2009 *Journal of AHIMA*.

Impact on Productivity and Accuracy

For a period of time, productivity and accuracy may suffer, as people become familiar with using the new coding systems. Questions to consider during this period:

- Will the increased number of codes impact the coding error rate?
- Will the increased number of codes impact the ability to detect errors?
- How will coding productivity be affected?
- Will decreased accuracy and productivity be limited to the transition period (or learning curve) with improved accuracy and productivity occurring in the long-term, due to the increased specificity of the codes?
- How long is the learning curve expected to be?
- How long will it take for coders to achieve proficiency or at least a proficiency level equal to before ICD-10-CM/PCS implementation?
- What will be the impact on quality of data during the learning curve?

Decreased coding accuracy will impact data quality. The length of this transition period, and the impact on data quality, will be less for ICD-10-CM than for ICD-10-PCS due to the similarities to ICD-9-CM.

Ultimately, it is expected that coding errors will decrease to a level below ICD-9-CM because of the improved logic and standardized definitions in ICD-10-PCS, the more accurate clinical terms in ICD-10-CM, and the more specific code descriptions in both systems. In the long-term, ICD-10-CM/PCS will fit more easily into the electronic health record environment, allowing more sophisticated computer-assisted coding technologies and advances in mapping from clinical terminologies, thus improving productivity and accuracy.

Other countries have reported, based on their ICD-10 implementation experience, that an initial productivity decline with gradual improvement over three to six months can be expected. Implementation variables that can affect productivity are the amount and level of dedicated preparation, program management, interdisciplinary team participation, extent of coder education and credentials, coder experience and understanding of anatomy and disease processes, extent of training, documentation status, and organization size and complexity.

Impact on Information Systems

Information Systems (IS) personnel will need to be oriented on the specifications of the code sets that they will need to know to implement systems changes, including the logic and hierarchical structure of ICD-10-CM/PCS. All electronic transactions requiring a diagnosis and/or procedure code will need to be reviewed (and possibly changed). Some of the various systems that will need to be reviewed include EHR systems, test-ordering systems, pharmacy systems, clinical reminder systems, billing systems, accounting and financial systems, registration and scheduling systems, advance beneficiary software, decision support systems, clinical systems, encoding software, medical necessity software, DRG and other PPS groupers, health record abstracting systems, case-mix systems, aggregate data reporting, utilization and quality management systems, clinical protocols, performance measurement systems, case management, disease management systems, provider profiling systems, compliance checking systems, medical necessity software, DRG groupers, claim submission systems, registries, state reporting systems, patient assessment data sets (for example, MDS, PAI, OASIS), managed care reporting system (HEDIS), and benefits determination.

Software will need to be developed to accommodate field size expansion, alphanumeric codes, redefinitions of code values, edit and logic changes, modifications of table structure, and expansion of flat files containing diagnosis codes and systems interfaces. Some specific examples include:

- Any field that requires a code will need to accommodate up to seven characters rather than five.
- Any field that requires a code will need to be changed to accept alphanumeric codes in addition to numeric codes. (This may not be an issue because of the V codes and E codes already used in ICD-9-CM.)

- ICD-10-CM codes may have up to four characters (numbers or letters) after the decimal point. In ICD-9-CM, there is a maximum of only two numbers after the decimal point. All ICD-10-PCS codes contain seven characters and alpha or numeric characters may appear in any position.
- The size of data fields accommodating descriptions of the codes may have to be reviewed. Code titles are much more descriptive and thus longer in ICD-10-CM than in ICD-9-CM.
- ICD-10-CM/PCS offers many more codes than ICD-9-CM. Therefore, the hardware will need to be able to accommodate additional data. Both ICD-9-CM and ICD-10-CM/PCS will have to be supported by the computer hardware.
- ICD-10-CM codes that consist of five characters may be confused with HCPCS Level II codes, which also begin with an alphabetic character. This will not be a problem if the decimal point is placed in the ICD-10-CM codes, but it might be a problem if the software did not use the decimal.

Additional consideration should be given to complete redefinition of code values and their interpretation, longer code descriptions, edit and logic changes, modifications of table structures, expansion of flat files containing diagnosis codes, and systems interfaces. It will also be necessary to determine the length of time that both legacy and new coding systems will need to be supported and address any system storage capacity issues. Reports and forms may require redesign or modification, and data mapping issues should be addressed.

Budgetary implications for hardware/software is a large part of IS planning and it is important to work with various vendors to determine when upgrades will be provided and if these are covered by any existing contracts. Consideration should be given to any contract renewals and future contract negotiations.

Impact on Budgeting and Reimbursement

There are several considerations in planning the budget for this transition. Various components of the implementation (costs of systems, hardware, software, and education) may be appropriated from different departmental budgets. It is also advantageous to spread the costs out over the timeline, rather than allocating all of the funds into one or two years, allowing for the absorption of the costs. During the implementation, increased out-sourced services may be required. It will be necessary to allocate time and resources to training, thus increased staffing needs related to productivity and accuracy, either short- or long-term, may be additional costs required. Further consulting services may be needed for backlogs, monitoring coding accuracy, or other support. Once again, this can be allocated over a several year timeframe.

Several training issues need to be addressed with billing and accounting personnel. The chief financial officer (CFO) of the organization will need to look at capital expenditures such as new or upgraded hardware, new software, training costs for coding professionals and other personnel, and the hiring of information systems personnel to accomplish the changeover.

In addition, there will likely be delays in payments from third-party payers until coders and billing personnel are fully trained on the system. Moreover, there may be increased numbers of claims denials or rejections due to inadequate coding, reporting, and processing.

Initially, payments should not be substantially affected from the standpoint of reimbursement systems. The General Equivalence Mappings (GEMs) files (discussed in detail in Chapter 5) are mappings designed to provide all sectors of the healthcare industry that use coded data with a tool to convert and test systems, link data in long-term clinical studies, develop application-specific mappings, and analyze data collected during the transition period and beyond. At some point, managed care contracts and negotiated rate schedules will be recalculated using ICD-10-CM/PCS data.

Eventually, ICD-10-CM/PCS data will allow appropriate refinements of reimbursement systems to better reflect the actual cost of patient care; will improve providers' and payers' ability to negotiate reimbursement rates; improve payers' ability to forecast the healthcare needs and analyze healthcare costs; reduce payers' and providers' costs due to improved ability to effectively monitor service and resource utilization, analyze healthcare costs, monitor outcomes, measure performance, and detect fraud and abuse. Moreover, the increased specificity will reduce the number of requests for medical records to justify payment because the increased detail and specificity in the ICD-10-CM/PCS codes should provide the information needed.

Chapter 5
Mapping and Legacy Data

The transition to new code sets means that data encoded in either the old (ICD-9-CM) or new (ICD-10-CM/PCS) code sets will need to be converted or translated to the other code set to preserve the informational value of healthcare data, regardless of whether it was collected before or after the transition to ICD-10-CM/PCS. Maps are an integral component of this data conversion or translation process.

Maps and How Are They Used

The process of mapping has been described as follows:

- Mapping is the process of creating one-way links between concepts and terms for specific purposes, often involving patient, administrative, or interface contexts:
  - Between concepts in reference terminology and external administrative or reimbursement classifications
  - Between concepts in reference terminology and interface terms/codes
  - Between concepts in different source terminologies or application vocabularies

- The one-way links can be through representation synonymy, term association, relationships, attributes, layers of granularity, composition/decomposition, and such.
- The result is a universal cross-reference map accounting for all concepts and terms.

Maps are created for many purposes, including exchange of data for patient care purposes, access to longitudinal data, reimbursement, epidemiology, public health data reporting, and reporting to regulators and state data organizations. A map's purpose is known as its use case.

Correct mapping requires a complete understanding of how data will be used. A function requirement, guideline, or use case is required to ensure that maps will be consistent across the application of all data. Use cases are a common methodology for establishing maps. A use case "defines the intended use, audience, and shared understanding of the target and source—key to development of a useful and reproducible map."

General Equivalence Mappings

Authoritative, detailed bidirectional mappings, referred to as General Equivalence Mappings (GEMs), have been developed between ICD-9-CM and ICD-10-CM/PCS. These mappings were developed with stakeholder input into their creation and maintenance, and discussed at public meetings of the ICD-9-CM Coordination and Maintenance Committee. The CDC developed the bidirectional mappings between the ICD-9-CM diagnosis codes and ICD-10-CM. CMS developed the bidirectional mappings between the ICD-9-CM procedure codes and ICD-10-PCS. The mappings are bidirectional because they include both backward and forward mappings. Mapping from ICD-10-CM/PCS back to ICD-9-CM is referred to as backward mapping. Mapping from ICD-9-CM to ICD-10-CM/PCS is referred to as forward mapping.

The CDC and CMS created the GEMs to ensure that consistency in national data is maintained. They have made a commitment to update the GEMs annually during the transition period prior to ICD-10-CM/PCS implementation and to maintain them for at least three years beyond the October 1, 2013, ICD-10-CM/PCS compliance date.

The GEMs were developed as a tool to assist with the conversion of ICD-9-CM codes to ICD-10-CM/PCS codes and vice versa. Since the GEMs need to support all uses of coded healthcare data, they were designed as a starting point, presenting all plausible translation alternatives.

The GEMs are a comprehensive translation dictionary that can be used to accurately and effectively translate large amounts of data from one code set to the other. The GEMs can be used to convert multiple databases from ICD-9-CM to ICD-10-CM/PCS, including payment systems, payment and coverage edits, risk adjustment logic, quality measures, disease management programs, financial modeling, and a variety of research applications involving trend data.

GEMs are *Not* Crosswalks

There is no simple crosswalk from ICD-9-CM to ICD-10-CM/PCS in the GEM files. A mapping that forces a simple correspondence—each ICD-9-CM code mapped only once—from the smaller, less detailed ICD-9-CM to the larger, more detailed ICD-10-CM/PCS defeats the purpose of upgrading to ICD-10-CM/PCS. It obscures the differences between the two code sets and eliminates any possibility of benefiting from the improvement in data quality that ICD-10-CM/PCS offer. Instead of a simple crosswalk, the GEM files attempt to organize those differences in a meaningful way, by linking a code to all valid alternatives in the other code set from which choices can be made depending on the use to which the code is put.

There is not a one-to-one match between ICD-9-CM and ICD-10-CM/PCS, for a variety of reasons including:

- There are new concepts in ICD-10-CM/PCS that are not present in ICD-9-CM
- For a small number of codes, there is no matching code in the GEMs
- More than one ICD-9-CM may be a possible translation of a given ICD-10-CM/PCS code
- More than one ICD-9-CM code may be required to convey the complete meaning of a given ICD-10-CM/PCS code
- A single ICD-9-CM code may map to multiple ICD-10-CM/PCS codes

If ICD-9-CM and ICD-10-CM/PCS were so similar that each term in ICD-9-CM could be mapped to an equivalent term in ICD-10-CM/PCS, there would not be any reason to switch to the new code sets.

GEMs Principles

The GEMs were designed to suggest, given a code in the source system (code set of origin in the mapping; the set being mapped *from*), as many possible alternatives in the target system (destination code set in the mapping; the set being mapped *to*) as are expressed or implied by that source system code. The GEMs follow five basic principles:

1. *Complete Code Definition*

   The complete meaning of a code is taken into account: the code description, all index entries that refer to the code, all includes notes, and all applicable *Coding Clinic* entries.

2. *Mapping Rules*

   If a code in the source system has no clear alternative in the target system, it is mapped to a target system code or codes according to a mapping rule, for example:

   > For ICD-10-PCS coronary artery body part values, "number of sites" treated must be mapped to ICD-9-CM codes specifying "number of vessels" treated. Although these two concepts are not equivalent, for mapping purposes "number of sites" in ICD-10-PCS is equal to "number of vessels" in ICD-9-CM.

3. *Mapping Specificity*
   Target system choices for a mapping entry are determined by the level of detail in the source system code.
4. *ICD-10-CM/PCS Detail*
   Where an ICD-10-CM/PCS code contains less detail than an ICD-9-CM code, the mapping assumes that the decision to reduce coded detail was consciously made, and that the detail omitted is obsolete or otherwise inapplicable.
5. *ICD-10-CM/PCS Improvements*
   Where an axis of classification between the two code sets is incompatible, the mapping assumes that the ICD-10-CM/PCS axis of classification is preferred.

The diagnosis and procedure GEMs use the same method and format. They consist of two mappings for the diagnosis codes and two mappings for the procedure codes: one in which ICD-9-CM is the source system and one in which ICD-10-CM or ICD-10-PCS is the source system.

Maps between ICD-9-CM and ICD-10-CM/PCS are an attempt to express relationships between the code sets that are more or less equivalent, insofar as this is possible. Because ICD-10-PCS and ICD-9-CM are so different, a map between them often presents only a series of possible compromises rather than the mirror image of a code in the other code set. The correlation between codes in ICD-10-CM and ICD-9-CM is close in some areas, and since the two code sets share the same conventions of organization and formatting, translating between them is straightforward. Many infectious disease, neoplasm, eye, and ear codes are examples of somewhat straightforward correspondence between the two code sets. In other areas—obstetrics, for example—whole chapters are organized along a different axis of classification. In such cases, translating between them most of the time can offer only a series of possible compromises rather than the mirror image of one code in the other code set.

Because the GEMs are general reference mappings, all reasonable equivalents are included, based on the particulars of the code in the source system. Due to the differences between ICD-9-CM and ICD-10-CM/PCS, a diagnosis or procedure code in ICD-9-CM may not have a close correspondent in ICD-10-CM/PCS. What this means for the GEMs is that in many cases, the code in the source system is linked to more than one alternative in the target system. For example, the single ICD-9-CM procedure code for suture of artery is linked to 195 ICD-10-PCS codes.

In the suture of artery scenario, the difference between the two code sets lies in the level of specificity. However, in ICD-10-CM, there are whole areas reclassified using different clinical emphases. In these cases, where the codes in the two code sets are not alike along an entire axis of classification, and where an all-inclusive mapping would contain an overwhelming and indiscriminate number of entries, rules were developed to link groups of codes in a consistent manner. Obstetrics diagnosis codes are a clear example. In ICD-9-CM, the patient is classified by diagnosis in relation to the

episode of care. In ICD-10-CM the patient is classified by diagnosis in relation to the patient's stage of
pregnancy. The GEM rules applied to linking these
diagnosis codes are shown in table 5.1.

**Figure 5.1. GEM rules applied to linking
diagnosis codes**

ICD-9-CM Source	ICD-10-CM Target	ICD-10-CM Source	ICD-9-CM Target
Unspecified episode of care	Unspecified trimester	Unspecified trimester	Unspecified episode of care
Antepartum	First trimester Second trimester Third trimester	First trimester	Antepartum
Delivered	Childbirth	Second trimester	Antepartum
Delivered with postpartum complication	Complication of puerperium	Third trimester	Antepartum
Postpartum complication	Complication of puerperium	Childbirth	Delivered
---	---	Complication of puerperium	Postpartum complication

In some cases, more than one code in the target
system may be required to fully represent a single
code in the source system. Following are two examples from the ICD-10-PCS mappings.

ICD-9-CM to ICD-10-PCS mapping:

"Laparoscopic salpingo-oophorectomy, bilateral"

ICD-9-CM Source	≈	ICD-10-PCS Target
65.63 Laparoscopic removal of both ovaries and tubes at same operative episode	≈	0UT24ZZ Resection of bilateral ovaries, percutaneous endoscopic approach AND 0UT74ZZ Resection of bilateral fallopian tubes, percutaneous endoscopic approach

ICD-10-PCS to ICD-9-CM mapping:

"Percutaneous Transluminal Coronary Angioplasty (PTCA) of two coronary arteries, with insertion of two coronary stents"

ICD-10-PCS Source	≈	ICD-9-CM Target
02713DZ Dilation of coronary artery, two sites using intraluminal device, percutaneous approach	≈	00.66 PTCA or coronary atherectomy AND 00.41 Procedure on two vessels AND 00.46 Insertion of two vascular stents AND 36.06 Insertion of non-drug-eluting coronary artery stents

The correspondence between codes in the source and target systems is approximate in most cases, which means no one code in the target system or linked combination of codes in the target system expresses the same essential meaning as the code in the source system. The difference between the two systems is typically in level of detail between the codes, and in nearly all cases the ICD-10-CM/PCS code is more detailed than the ICD-9-CM code. As with translating between languages, translating between coding systems does not necessarily yield an exact match. Context is key and the specific purpose of an applied mapping must be identified before the most appropriate option can be selected. The GEMs together provide a general (many-to-many) reference mapping that can be refined to fit the requirements of an applied mapping.

A code in the source system may be used multiple times in the GEM, each time linked to a different code in the target system. This is because the GEM contains alternative equivalent relationships from which the appropriate applied mapping can be selected.

The diagnosis and procedure GEMs use the same method and format. They consist of two mappings for the diagnosis codes and two mappings for the procedure codes: one in which ICD-9-CM is the source system and one in which ICD-10-CM/PCS is the source system in the following table.

Diagnosis Code Set			Procedure Code Set		
Source (from)	Target (to)	AKA	Source (from)	Target (to)	AKA
ICD-9-CM	ICD-10-CM	diagnosis forward mapping	ICD-9-CM	ICD-10-PCS	procedure forward mapping
ICD-10-CM	ICD-9-CM	diagnosis backward mapping	ICD-10-PCS	ICD-9-CM	procedure backward mapping

The GEMs are complete in their description of all the mapping possibilities as well as when there are new concepts in ICD-10-CM that are not found in ICD-9-CM. All ICD-9-CM codes and all ICD-10-CM/PCS codes are included in the collective GEMs:

- All ICD-10-CM codes are in the ICD-10-CM to ICD-9-CM GEM.
- All ICD-9-CM diagnosis codes are in the ICD-9-CM to ICD-10-CM GEM.
- All ICD-10-PCS codes are in the ICD-10-PCS to ICD-9-CM GEM.
- All ICD-9-CM procedure codes are in the ICD-9-CM to ICD-10-PCS GEM.

There are GEMs for more than 99 percent of all ICD-10-CM codes and for 100 percent of the ICD-10-PCS codes. In 0.6 percent of the ICD-10-CM codes, there are no similar codes in ICD-9-CM to which the ICD-10-CM code could be mapped because these ICD-10-CM codes represent new diagnosis concepts that were introduced in ICD-10-CM and do not exist in ICD-9-CM. For example, there are codes for blood type and underdosing in ICD-10-CM, but there are no comparable concepts in ICD-9-CM.

For any particular code in the source system in a GEM, all reasonable code translation alternatives are included in the respective GEM, based on the complete meaning of the code in the source system. For example, in the ICD-9-CM to ICD-10-CM GEM, all reasonable translation alternatives are included for a particular ICD-9-CM code (the code in the source system), based on the complete meaning of the ICD-9-CM code. The complete meaning of a code includes tabular instructions, index entries, official coding guidelines, and applicable advice from *Coding Clinic for ICD-9-CM*. There may be multiple translation alternatives for a source system code, all of which are equally plausible. This is true of both the ICD-10-CM/PCS to ICD-9-CM GEMs and the ICD-9-CM to ICD-10-CM/PCS GEMs.

Using the GEMs

The GEMs were designed as a general purpose translation tool for all types of providers, payers, and other users of coded data. The translations are based on the meaning of the code as contained in the tabular instructions, index entries, official coding guidelines, and applicable *Coding Clinic for ICD-9-CM* advice. They were developed independently without reference to Medicare data. Their applicability extends equally to all types of users— including providers, payers, researchers, and application development vendors. The GEMs are free of charge and in the public domain.

The GEMs were designed principally to give all sectors of the industry a common starting point from which to either: (1) convert their ICD-9-CM-based applications to native ICD-10-CM/PCS based applications that use ICD-10-CM/PCS codes directly, or (2) to create applied mappings in either direction—ICD-10-CM/PCS back to ICD-9-CM or ICD-9-CM forward to ICD-10-CM/PCS. These can be "one-to-one" or "one-to-many" mappings, depending on the use to which the mapping is put.

The GEMs are not biased toward any particular use, but are based on the meaning of the code in the source system.

Converting an ICD-9-CM based application to a native ICD-10-CM/PCS version of the same application is indicated when:

- The application analyzes coded records in a series of defined steps and decisions are made based on logical relationships between the codes.
- The application will be an ongoing part of systems that use ICD-10-CM/PCS codes after implementation.
- ICD-10-CM/PCS coded data collected from the application after implementation will be used to make decisions for future application changes or new application design.
- It has been determined that the results using an ICD-10-CM/PCS to ICD-9-CM one-to-one mapping are unacceptable.

The GEMs will not necessarily be used for every data conversion project. When a small number of ICD-9-CM codes are being converted to ICD-10-CM/PCS codes, it may be quicker, easier, and more accurate to simply look up the codes in an ICD-10-CM/PCS book or encoder.

Maps between ICD-9-CM and ICD-10-CM/PCS should not be used for coding individual medical records. Mapping is not the same as coding. Mapping links concepts in two code sets without consideration of patient medical record information. Coding involves the assignment of the most appropriate code based on medical record documentation and applicable coding rules and guidelines.

Linking Coded Data

It is important to understand the kinds of differences that need to be reconciled in linking coded data. The method used to reconcile those differences may vary, depending on whether the data is used for research, claims adjudication, or analyzing coding patterns between the two code sets; whether the desired outcome is to present an all-embracing look at the possibilities (one-to-many mapping) or to offer the one "best" compromise for the application (one-to-one mapping); whether the desired outcome is to translate existing coded data to their counterparts in the new code set (forward mapping) or to track newly coded data back to what they may have been in the previous code set (backward mapping); or any number of other factors. The scope of the differences varies, is complex, and cannot be overlooked if quality mapping and useful coded data are the desired outcomes.

Applied Mappings

It would be impossible to produce a "one-size-fits-all" set of mappings because a mapping is heavily dependent on its purpose. For example, a map for reimbursement uses different rules and contains different entries than a map for research.

Creating a one-to-one applied mapping for a specific purpose is indicated when:

- The current application cannot be converted to process ICD-10-CM/PCS codes directly.
  - Application or platform limitations
  - Financial constraints
- The current application is being replaced by a new application on or shortly after ICD-10-CM/PCS implementation.
- The current application does not organize codes into lists.

While the GEMs are not themselves applied mappings, the GEMs are the foundation upon which applied mappings can readily be built. In addition, the process for creating applied mappings, with the GEMs as the starting point, can be used and reused in converting similar systems or applications from ICD-9-CM to ICD-10-CM/PCS. The GEMs together provide a general (many-to-many) reference mapping that can be refined to fit the requirements of an applied mapping. For a particular code entry, the GEM may contain several possible translations, each on a separate row. The code in the source system is listed on a new row as many times as there are alternatives in the target system. Each correspondence is formatted as a code pair. The user must choose from among the alternatives a single code in the target system if a one-to-one mapping is desired.

Applied mappings can resolve mapping conflicts and narrow the possible choices in the target code set by implementing a set of user-defined criteria. The GEMs can be refined based on the purpose, or use case, of the map, whether the map is being used to map to a grouper in the old code set, to track clinical data over time for research purposes, or to check on the effectiveness of a facility's quality improvement measures.

- An applied mapping for reimbursement would not require a precise match between the code sets, but only that the code in question be assigned to the same reimbursement group as a comparable code in the target code set.
- An applied mapping to track codes for clinical studies would allow the user to narrow the possible choices to the level of detail in the codes around which the study was designed. This is sometimes called a "*best map*" and can differ depending on whether the study was designed in ICD-9-CM and mapping forward or in ICD-10-CM/PCS and mapping backward.

An applied mapping for quality improvement may be most useful if it includes the highest level of detail possible, regardless of the direction of the map. This will allow the most information to be examined about the patient's condition and the procedures performed, if the most detailed codes available from both code sets can be included, based on the documentation in the medical record.

Use Cases

Use cases are required to ensure that maps will be consistent across the application of all the data. The development of the use case should be as complete as possible. Questions that should be asked when developing use cases are:

- How will the mapped data be used? Will it be used for reimbursement, research, outcome measurements, or public health studies?
- How will the data be transmitted and to what systems?
- Will the data be used for picklists?
- Will prompts be implemented based on the map?
- Will the mapped data be categorized, classified, or grouped into other data sets?
- Will the data be stored? If yes, how will it be stored?

The map's use case is the core upon which the guidelines and heuristics, or rules, for creating the map are specified. Guidelines and heuristics must be very detailed, because all maps must be reproducible, meaning that once a map has been created, others not involved in the creation of the map should be able to verify the map's accuracy by reproducing the map following its guidelines and heuristics.

Where the GEMs give all plausible meanings of a source system code in the target system, an applied map must choose the one closest match for the source system code. Depending on the use case of the map, the choice of closest match may differ. Rules specific to the applied mapping should be developed to promote consistency and document the decisions made.

Examples of Uses for Applied Mappings

An example of a situation when the selected code in the target system might differ depending on the use case of the applied mapping is found throughout the codes in the ICD-9-CM and ICD-10-CM obstetrics chapters. For an ICD-10-CM code specifying placenta previa in a third trimester patient, the ICD-10-CM to ICD-9-CM GEMs entry is:

O44.03 Placenta previa specified as without hemorrhage, third trimester

Translates to

641.01 Placenta previa without hemorrhage, with delivery
641.03 Placenta previa without hemorrhage, antepartum

The two ICD-9-CM translations obviously say two different things. One says that the patient delivered on this encounter, the other says this is an antepartum encounter. Since the ICD-10-CM code does not specify encounter information in the code description, both translations are equally correct. An applied mapping must choose the one closest match from ICD-10-CM/PCS to ICD-9-CM based on the needs of the application.

There is only one way to refine this entry for a clinically accurate ICD-10-CM to ICD-9-CM applied mapping: to choose among the alternatives in ICD-9-CM, the user must have access to the detail in the original record. If the patient record is not available, or the mapping application is intended to establish general rules for translation rather than deciding on a case-by-case basis, then a consistent method must be derived and documented for resolving the disparity in classification between the two systems. Depending on the use case of the map, the user may want to equate all ICD-10-CM obstetric codes with ICD-9-CM codes indicating a particular episode of care and not include the other ICD-9-CM codes as alternatives in the ICD-10-CM to ICD-9-CM applied mapping.

In the placenta previa example, if the application is for hospital inpatient encounters, the closest match would most likely be:

O44.03 Placenta previa specified as without hemorrhage, third trimester

Mapped to

641.01 Placenta previa without hemorrhage, with delivery

If the application were used for outpatient and physician office encounters, the closest match would most likely be:

O44.03 Placenta previa specified as without hemorrhage, third trimester

Mapped to

641.03 Placenta previa without hemorrhage, antepartum

Mapping from ICD-9-CM to ICD-10-CM, however, would require that all ICD-9-CM codes be used. In this case, specific information from the patient record would be necessary to determine the correct trimester needed for the ICD-10-CM codes. If this level of detail were unavailable or unnecessary, a rule would need to be established for identifying a default trimester for purposes of an applied ICD-9-CM to ICD-10-CM mapping.

Another example is percutaneous transluminal coronary angioplasty (PTCA). ICD-9-CM and ICD-10-PCS classify the body part quite differently. ICD-9-CM classifies the body part by number of *vessels* treated, and ICD-10-PCS classifies by the number of *sites* treated regardless of the number of vessels. For example, a PTCA could treat two separate lesions along the same vessel. In ICD-10-PCS this is considered two sites for coding purposes, whereas in ICD-9-CM it is considered one vessel.

The ramification for mapping is that the ICD-10-PCS code indicating that four sites were treated must be linked to all ICD-9-CM code alternatives indicating the number of vessels treated, since all four sites could conceivably be on the same vessel. To determine the most clinically accurate code alternative, the user would need access to the detail in the original record. If the patient record is not available, or the mapping application is intended to establish general rules for translation rather than deciding on a case-by-case basis, then a consistent method must be derived and documented for resolving the disparity in body part classification between the two systems. These kinds of decisions must take into account the specific applied mapping needed.

Depending on the mapping application, the user may want to equate vessels with sites or ignore the ICD-9-CM adjunct codes for number of vessels altogether in the applied mapping. These decisions require considering the ramifications of lost detail for accurate reimbursement and for transposing research data gathered in one system and converted to another.

An additional example of the types of decisions that need to be made in an applied mapping is ICD-9-CM procedure code 00.53, Implantation or replacement of cardiac resynchronization pacemaker pulse generator only. This code captures either an initial implantation or a replacement of a pacemaker pulse generator. In ICD-10-PCS, "replacement" is captured through a combination of removal and insertion codes. So, ICD-9-CM 00.53 maps to both the ICD-10-PCS codes for insertion of pacemaker pulse generator and combination entries for removal and insertion. To refine the mapping entry, first the user must decide whether or not the applied mapping is going to encompass both the single and combination translation. This decision depends on the mapping application.

These examples demonstrate why a "one size fits all" crosswalk is not possible, and why applied maps based on the GEMs are the closest we are likely to come to an industry-wide consistent mapping standard.

The ICD-10-CM/PCS reimbursement mappings (discussed in more detail below) are a prominent example of an applied mapping.

Reimbursement Mappings

Reimbursement mappings were developed by CMS in response to non-Medicare industry requests for a "standard one-to-one reimbursement crosswalk," which is a temporary mechanism for mapping ICD-10-CM/PCS codes submitted on or after October 1, 2013, back to "reimbursement equivalent" ICD-9-CM codes.

The use of the reimbursement mapping would not provide the user with the ability of taking advantage of the significant increase in detail within ICD-10-CM/PCS. Whenever possible, use of the GEMs for mapping purposes is preferable.

CMS is not using the ICD-10-CM/PCS reimbursement mappings for any purpose. They are converting their systems and applications to accept ICD-10-CM/PCS codes directly.

Unlike the GEMs, which include all plausible translation alternatives for each code in a system, the reimbursement mappings offer a single recommended mapping of each ICD-10-CM/PCS code to a single ICD-9-CM alternative. The reimbursement mappings are one-to-one mappings in the sense that they choose a single ICD-9-CM translation among alternatives.

In order to develop the reimbursement mappings, CMS used the GEMs as a starting point by selecting the best ICD-9-CM code that maps to each ICD-10-CM/PCS code. The reimbursement mappings identify the best matching ICD-9-CM code that can be used for reimbursement purposes for each ICD-10-CM/PCS code. There are two

reimbursement mappings:
- ICD-10-CM to ICD-9-CM for diagnosis codes
- ICD-10-PCS to ICD-9-CM for procedure codes

All ICD-10-CM/PCS codes are in the reimbursement mappings; however, not all ICD-9-CM codes are in the reimbursement mappings. Certain ICD-9-CM codes use outmoded terminology or an axis of classification that has been replaced by something more clinically relevant in the ICD-10 code set. The inevitable result of a process that chooses a single ICD-9-CM code among alternatives is that the other ICD-9-CM alternatives are not included in the mapping.

The reimbursement mapping contains an entry for every ICD-10-CM/PCS code. However, not every ICD-9-CM code is used in the mapping. Certain ICD-9-CM codes use outmoded terminology or an axis of classification replaced by something more clinically relevant in the ICD-10-CM/PCS code sets. As a result, an ICD-10-CM/PCS code is mapped to the closest clinically relevant alternative ICD-9-CM code, or the most frequently used ICD-9-CM code, in the process outlined above. A process that chooses a single ICD-9-CM code among alternatives must of course leave the other ICD-9-CM alternatives unused.

Users of the reimbursement mapping may want to sort the mapping entries by ICD-9-CM code and determine if any particular ICD-9-CM codes used by their legacy systems (for example, those qualifying for carve-outs or other special treatment) are not mapped to. Such codes would no longer be used when input is coming to their legacy systems through the reimbursement mapping. If there are ICD-9-CM codes not used by the reimbursement mapping that are essential to the legacy system, then the reimbursement mapping can be modified for that system (which would then be another type of applied mapping).

Development of the Reimbursement Mappings

Where an ICD-10-CM/PCS code translates to more than one ICD-9-CM code, a single choice is required to create a functioning crosswalk. When the GEM offered more than one ICD-9-CM translation for an ICD-10-CM/PCS code, two reference data sources were queried to find the most frequently coded of the ICD-9-CM alternatives. These reference data sources were used to help select a single ICD-9-CM code among the translation alternatives. Medicare data were used in the form of approximately 11 million MedPAR records. All-payer data were represented by approximately four million inpatient hospital records available from the California Office of Statewide Health Planning and Development.

Both data sets come from hospital admission data, and choosing between ICD-9-CM alternatives may reflect frequencies more characteristic of inpatient than outpatient data when the two differ. An example of this can be found in the obstetrics codes specifying complications of pregnancy. Because ICD-10-CM does not specify encounter information, that is, whether the patient delivered during the encounter, the reimbursement mapping must choose between two ICD-9-CM alternatives, one that specifies antepartum encounter, the other a delivery. For inpatient hospital data, the ICD-9-CM codes specifying delivery are far more frequent, while in outpatient and physician data, one would expect the ICD-9-CM codes specifying antepartum encounter to dominate.

In the vast majority of cases, one ICD-9-CM alternative was clearly dominant. The dominant ICD-9-CM alternative was then chosen as the ICD-9-CM code for the reimbursement mapping. When the Medicare reference data set and the all-payer reference data set disagreed, the code with the highest Medicare frequency was chosen for nonobstetric, nonnewborn diagnoses and procedures. For obstetric and newborn diagnoses and procedures, the all-payer data set was given precedence.

When there were too few cases in either reference data set by itself, the two data sets were combined to achieve a higher frequency. Rule-based selection criteria and clinical judgment were used to select a mapping for the approximately 300 diagnosis and 120 procedure codes, which were so rarely recorded that the reference data sets were unable to identify a clear best alternative.

Reimbursement Mapping—Example
Following is an example of the process used to create the reimbursement mappings.

Reimbursement Mapping of Dominant ICD-9-CM Code Alternative

ICD-10-CM Code	ICD-9-CM Code Alternatives in the GEM	Med-PAR Records	Med-PAR %	Calif. Records	Calif. %	Re-imbursement Mapping
J45.22, Mild intermittent asthma with status asthmaticus	493.01, Extrinsic asthma with status asthmaticus 493.11, Intrinsic asthma with status asthmaticus	384 49	88% 11%	3604 32	99% 0%	X

If necessary, the reimbursement mappings may be used to process ICD-10-CM/PCS-based claims received on or after October 1, 2013, with a legacy ICD-9-CM-based system as part of a planned transition period, until systems and processes are developed to process ICD-10-CM/PCS-based claims directly.

Data Trending Challenges

Although good mappings will facilitate the process of translating between the old and new code sets, there will still be challenges in relating data coded under ICD-9-CM to data coded under ICD-10-CM/PCS due to the differences in the code sets. This would severely impact reports that compile statistical data for trend analysis. Such reports may be used for rating purposes, effectiveness of care, provider profiling, actuarial analysis, and such. Ad hoc reports used to track utilization review, immunizations, maternity, transplants, disease management, cost savings, and such will also be affected. Any activity involving comparisons of historical and current data, such as retrospective audits, would be impacted.

Flawed decisions may be made due to reliance on distorted, inaccurate, or misinterpreted data, and/or due to comparability problems between data reported in ICD-9-CM and that reported in ICD-10-CM/PCS. Caution should be exercised when interpreting longitudinal data, as diagnoses and procedures may be classified differently if the analysis crosses the transition timeframe.

The obstetric codes are an example of a data comparability issue. In ICD-9-CM, the obstetric conditions are classified according to episode of care, whereas in ICD-10-CM, they are classified according to the trimester in which the condition occurred.

Another example is open wounds. An ICD-9-CM code for "complicated open wound" is not easily translated to ICD-10-CM. The ICD-9-CM clinical concept "complicated" as it pertains to open wounds includes delayed healing, delayed treatment, foreign body, or infection. ICD-10-CM does not classify open wound codes based on the general concept "complicated." It categorizes open wounds by wound type—for example, laceration or puncture wound—and then further classifies each type of open wound according to whether a foreign body is present. ICD-10-CM open wound codes do not mention delayed healing or delayed treatment, and instructional notes advise the coder to code any associated infection separately. Therefore, there is no simple translation in ICD-10-CM for the complicated open wound concept in ICD-9-CM.

Some data comparability issues may not be apparent from the code descriptions themselves. For example, the acute myocardial infarction codes may look very comparable in ICD-9-CM and ICD-10-CM, but in fact, they are quite different because in ICD-9-CM, an acute myocardial infarction is one occurring within the past eight weeks, whereas in ICD-10-CM, it is defined as one occurring within the past four weeks.

Combination Codes Create Challenges

Situations when a combination code in one code set corresponds to two or more discrete codes in the other code set presents data comparability challenges because the combination code must be linked simultaneously to two or more codes in the other code set. Each discrete code is a partial expression of the information contained in the combination code and must be linked together to fully describe the same conditions or procedures specified in the combination code. For example, sometimes an ICD-10-PCS code must be linked to multiple ICD-9-CM codes because the ICD-9-CM primary procedure code is incomplete and so requires "adjunct" codes to convey specific information about the procedure. The detail contained in an ICD-9-CM primary procedure code and an ICD-9-CM adjunct code can be found in a single ICD-10-PCS code. An example would be a percutaneous transluminal coronary angioplasty (PTCA) of three coronary arteries, with insertion of three drug eluting stents. In the ICD-10-PCS to ICD-9-CM GEM, ICD-10-PCS code 027234Z, Dilation of coronary artery, three sites with drug-eluting intraluminal device, percutaneous approach, is mapped to a cluster of four ICD-9-CM codes that are needed to fully represent this procedure:

00.66 Percutaneous transluminal coronary angioplasty [PTCA] or coronary atherectomy

00.42 Procedure on three vessels

00.47 Insertion of three vascular stents

36.07 Insertion of drug-eluting coronary artery stents(s)

In the ICD-9-CM to ICD-10-PCS map, ICD-9-CM code 00.66 is mapped to ICD-10-PCS code 027234Z (as well as to all of the other ICD-10-PCS codes for dilation of coronary artery), but codes 00.42, 00.47, and 36.07 cannot be mapped to any ICD-10-PCS code because there is no comparable concept of an adjunct procedure in ICD-10-PCS.

Appendix A
ICD-10 Preparation Checklist

by Sue Bowman, RHIA, CCS, and Ann Zeisset, RHIT, CCS, CCS-P

Although the implementation date for ICD-10-CM and ICD-10-PCS (jointly referred to as "ICD-10" throughout the rest of this document) may still be several years away, it is not too early to begin planning for the transition, and even putting some of those plans in motion. A well-planned, well-managed implementation process will increase the chances of a smooth, successful transition. Experience in other countries has shown that early preparation is key to success. The best way to manage the challenges inherent in making a transition of this magnitude is to tackle them in a phased approach.

Some of the preparation activities necessary for implementation provide benefits to the organization even before ICD-10 is implemented, such as medical record documentation improvement

Source: Bowman, Sue, and Ann Zeisset. "ICD-10 Preparation Checklist" (Updated June 2007).

Editor's note: This article updates information contained in "ICD-10 Preparation Checklist, parts 1 and 2," originally published in the June and July-August 2004 issues of the Journal of AHIMA.

strategies and efforts to expand coding staff knowledge and skills. Also, an early start allows for resource allocation, such as costs for systems changes and education as well as staff time devoted to implementation processes, to be spread over several years. Thus, many of the costs can be absorbed by existing annual budgets rather than requiring a large budgetary investment at one time.

The following checklist and proposed phased approach to implementation were prepared to guide healthcare organizations in planning and managing the transition toward ICD-10.

Phase 1—Impact Assessment

The first stage of preparation involves assessing the impact of the change to new coding systems and identifying key tasks and objectives. Major tasks in this phase include creating an implementation planning team; identifying and budgeting for required information system (IS) changes; and assessing, budgeting, and implementing clinician and code set user education.

Target Audience
- Health information management (HIM) leadership team
- Coding professionals
- Senior management
- Medical staff
- Financial management (including accounting and billing personnel)
- IS personnel

- Clinical department managers
- Other data users (e.g., quality management, utilization management, case management, performance improvement, tumor registry, trauma registry, research)
- Vendors (contract coding, software developers)
- Business associates (including payers)

Goals

Organizationwide Implementation Strategy

1. Establish an interdisciplinary steering committee to oversee ICD-10 implementation.

   - The committee should include representation from HIM, including both an HIM services manager and a representative from the staff responsible for code assignment; senior management; medical staff; financial management; and IS.
   - The leader of this committee should serve as the project manager throughout the course of the implementation process; an HIM background would be advantageous for this role.
   - This project manager should serve as a positive change agent for ICD-10 implementation.
   - The steering committee would develop the organization's ICD-10 implementation strategy and identify the actions, persons responsible, and deadlines for the various tasks required to complete the transition. In addition, this plan should include estimated budget needs for each year leading up to implementation, as well as any

post-implementation budgetary issues (such as additional training needs or the need for contractors to assist with coding backlogs or resolution of identified post-implementation problems), for early financial planning.

- Conduct regularly scheduled standing meetings on a consistent basis to ensure communication among key stakeholders.

2. Create ICD-10 code set impact awareness throughout the organization.

- Educate senior management, IS personnel, clinical department managers, and medical staff on the coming transition to ICD-10 and the necessity for this transition (e.g., department managers' meetings, medical staff meetings, specialized meetings with senior management and IS).
- Educate senior management on:
  - value of new code sets
  - adoption and implementation process (including timeline)
  - preparation and transition effects on organizational operations (e.g., systems changes, processes, policies and procedures)
  - impact on coding productivity and accuracy
  - budgetary considerations
- Educate the organization's clinical department managers about the:
  - value of new code sets
  - expected timeline for approval and implementation
  - differences between ICD-10-CM and

      ICD-10-PCS and how each is used
- differences between legacy and new coding systems
- impact on each particular department and budgetary considerations

- Educate medical staff on:
  - value of new code sets
  - expected timeline for approval and implementation
  - differences between legacy and new coding systems
  - implementation plan and how it can be adapted for use in their own practices
  - impact on individual physicians and their budgetary considerations
  - impact on documentation practices and the importance of a strategy for documentation improvement

- Once the notice of proposed rule-making (NPRM) is published that establishes the timeline and expected implementation date, educate all of the above on key provisions of this rule.

3.   Employ change management strategies to minimize "fear of change" factor.

4.   Assess organizational readiness for data standard changes, considering the impact on:
- Affected staff
- Information systems (affected systems, applications, databases)
- Documentation process and work flow

- Data availability and use
- Organizational capacity (including budget)

5. HIM managers and coding professionals should:
   - Educate themselves on the benefits and value of ICD-10—particularly within the context of national healthcare data quality measurement initiatives.
   - Understand the regulatory process for adoption, anticipated implementation timeline and variables affecting the timeline, and the ICD-10 implementation process so they can facilitate discussions, answer questions, and act as a resource for others.
   - Learn how ICD-10 fits within the overall electronic health record (EHR), the nationwide health information network (NHIN), and data quality initiatives.
   - Learn the structure, organization, and unique features of ICD-10-CM and ICD-10-PCS and gain a moderate level of familiarity with the coding systems. Methods include, but are not limited to:
     - Attending educational sessions
       . audio conferences
       . convention presentations
       . local conference presentations
       . online training
     - Reading *Journal of AHIMA* and other pertinent publications, including but not limited to:
       . Pertinent feature articles

- . "Word from Washington" columns
- . E-alerts
- . E-HIM® Fundamentals columns
- . AHIMA Practice Briefs
- . CodeWrite newsletter
- . ICD-10 educational materials, such as the AHIMA book *ICD-10-CM and ICD-10-PCS Preview*
- Reviewing ICD-10 materials on Centers for Medicare & Medicaid Services (CMS) and National Center for Health Statistics (NCHS) Web sites:
  - . ICD-10-CM coding guidelines
  - . ICD-10-PCS reference manual
  - . Documentation and User's Guide for the general equivalence map between ICD-10-PCS and ICD-9-CM
- Participating in the AHIMA ICD-10 Implementation Community of Practice (CoP) (limited to AHIMA members).
- Monitoring the ICD-10 page of the AHIMA Web site, AHIMA HIPAA CoP, and AHIMA Coding CoP for important news and other relevant information (limited to AHIMA members).
- Reading the 2003 report "ICD-10-Field Testing Project, Report on Findings: Perceptions, Ideas, and Recommendations from Coding Professionals Across the Nation" by the American Hospital Association (AHA) and AHIMA in the FORE Library: HIM Body of Knowledge (BoK).

- Staying abreast of news/announcements provided by AHIMA in order to keep up-to-date on status of adoption/implementation.

6. Develop a budget for ICD-10 implementation.
   - Identify the specific departmental budget(s) that will be responsible for the cost of systems changes, hardware and software upgrades, and education.
   - Determine whether there will be a need for increased staffing or consulting services to assist with IS changes, coding backlogs, monitoring of coding accuracy, or to support other aspects of implementation.
   - Total implementation costs should be allocated over a several year time frame to allow for the absorption of the costs.

7. Conduct a detailed assessment of staff education needs (for all staff) and determine budgetary estimates.
   - Identify educational needs of staff and determine the following:
     - Who needs education?
     - What type and level of education do they need?
   - The multiple categories of users of coded data require varying levels of education on the new coding systems. These categories of users include:
     - Coding professionals

- Other HIM staff responsible for health record services
- Billing
- Accounting
- Corporate compliance office
- Auditors and/or consultants performing documentation or coding review
- Clinicians
- Clinical department managers
- Quality management
- Utilization management
- Patient access and registration (if they are involved in medical necessity determinations)
- Ancillary departments
- Data quality management staff
- Data security personnel
- Data analysts working both inside and outside the organization
- Researchers
- Other data users (e.g., performance improvement)
- IS personnel
- Prepaid contract managers and negotiators
- Determine the best method, in terms of a balance between effectiveness and cost, of providing education. There are numerous methods of providing education today, such as:
    - traditional face-to-face classroom teaching
    - audio conferences
    - CD-ROM or downloadable materials (self directed learning)
    - Various forms of Web-based instruction (self-directed or instructor-led)

- Determine whether education will be provided through internal or external mechanisms, or both.

8. Evaluate current data flow, work flows, and operational processes to identify processes and reports that will be affected and determine opportunities for improvement.

9. Assess extent of changes to systems, processes, policies/procedures, and education needs; determine associated budgetary assessments and compare to initial budget estimates and make note of variances for planning purposes.

10. Assess impact on organizational operations of change to new coding systems, such as implementation costs beyond the investment associated with education and systems changes; this would provide an assessment of the total cost of ownership for this change.
    - Assess loss of code assignment and claims submission productivity during the learning curve period for users of code sets.
    - Educate data users (e.g., case management, utilization management, quality management, data analysts) on data comparability issues and impact on longitudinal data analysis.
    - Educate data users on differences in classification of diseases and procedures in the new coding systems, including definitions

and code category composition, in order to assess impact on data trends.

11. Assess status of payers' and other business associates' progress toward ICD-10 preparedness by confirming when they expect to be ready.

12. Provide senior management with regular updates as to project status.

13. Keep affected staff informed through frequent updates regarding progress, next steps, and issue identification and resolution.

Information Systems

1. Orient IS personnel on the specifications of the code sets that they will need to know to implement systems changes, including the logic and hierarchical structure of ICD-10-CM and ICD-10-PCS. The following questions should be addressed:
   - What is the character-length specification for ICD-10-CM and ICD-10-PCS codes?
   - Is it alphabetic, numeric, or a combination of both?
   - Are the alphabetic characters case-sensitive?
   - Does the code format include a decimal?
   - Can codes, descriptions, and applicable support documentation and guidelines be obtained in a machine-readable form?
   - What coding systems will it replace and when will it replace them?

- Are forward and backward maps available
  between the legacy and new coding systems? If
  so what is the defined use case for each?
- How many data management systems will be
  affected and what types of systems changes
  will need to be made? (see list of specific
  examples under no. 2 below)

2. Perform a comprehensive systems audit for
   ICD-10 compatibility
   - Inventory all databases and systems appli-
     cations that use ICD-9-CM codes, giving
     consideration to:
     - Use of application service provider vs.
       internally developed system interface and
       other affected software programs
     - How are ICD-9-CM codes used in each
       system? Will ICD-10-CM or ICD-10-PCS
       codes serve the same purpose and will a
       change in code sets impact the results?
     - Where do the codes come from (e.g.,
       manually entered versus imported from
       another system)?
     - How quality of data is checked
     - Interfaces between systems
   - Map electronic data flow to inventory all
     reports that contain ICD-9-CM codes.
   - Perform a detailed analysis of systems
     changes that need to occur. Prioritize
     sequence of systems changes and estimate
     cost of changes. Refine previous budgetary
     estimates as necessary.
     - Determine required software changes:

. Field size expansion
. Change to alphanumeric composition
. Use of decimals
. Complete redefinition of code values and their interpretation
. Longer code descriptions
. Edit and logic changes
. Modifications of table structures
. Expansion of flat files containing diagnosis codes
. Systems interfaces
- Assess changes to the various systems and applications that use coded data will need to be made, including:
. EHR systems
. Decision support systems
. Billing systems
. Clinical systems
. Encoding software
. Computer-assisted coding applications
. Medical record abstracting systems
. Registration and scheduling systems
. Aggregate data reporting
. Utilization management
. Quality management systems
. Case mix systems
. Accounting systems
. Case management systems
. Disease management systems
. Provider profiling systems
. Clinical protocols
. Test ordering systems
. Clinical systems

- Clinical reminder systems
- Performance measurement systems
- Medical necessity software
- Determine length of time both legacy and new coding systems will need to be supported and whether system storage capacity will need to be increased. Types of support to be considered include:
  - Systems vendors—is support for both legacy and new coding systems addressed in the contract? How long is support for both coding systems anticipated? What kind of support is needed?
  - Internal IS department—how long will the ICD-9 coding system continue to be accessible and to whom will it be accessible (e.g., data analysis personnel may require access for a longer period of time than the coding or billing staff)? Is system storage capacity adequate or will it need to be increased?
  - Data users—how long will legacy data need to be available for data analysis, research, etc.?
  - Billing—legacy system will still be needed for old claims and re-bills.
  - Coding professionals—knowledge of both coding systems will continue to be needed.
- Determine which reports will require modification of format or layout.
- Determine which forms will require redesign.
- Conduct a data mapping overview.
- Identify new or upgraded hardware/software requirements and determine budgetary

implications (e.g., larger computer monitors, more powerful hard drive)

- If the coding process is currently manual (use of hard-copy code books), consideration should be given to using electronic tools (such as an encoder) when ICD-10 is implemented, which will result in additional hardware and software requirements; although it would be technically possible for coding professionals to use a paper-based version of ICD-10, given the size and structure of these systems, they would be easiest to use in an electronic format.
- Will hardware upgrades be needed to ensure optimal system performance?

3. Determine vendor readiness and timelines for upgrading software to new coding systems and determine if upgrades are covered by any existing contracts.

- Communicate with vendors of software that incorporates ICD codes to determine when upgrades reflecting the new coding systems will be ready and whether any cost for the upgrades will be passed on to the organization, and if so, the projected cost and in what year it will be incurred.
- If necessary, include costs of upgrade in ICD-10 budget.
- Contract renewals
- Determine the anticipated timeline for testing the performance of the new code sets in your systems environment.

- Work with vendors to coordinate installation of new or upgraded software.
- Actively participate in any vendor user group meetings regarding ICD-10 implementation.

4. Build flexibility into systems currently under development to ensure ICD-10 and, when possible, the next version of ICD compatibility.

Education of Coding Professionals

1. Assess adequacy of staff knowledge and skills for translation of clinical data into codes for secondary use.
   - Evaluate coding personnel's baseline knowledge in skills to identify knowledge gaps in the areas of medical terminology, anatomy and physiology, pathophysiology, and pharmacology. Measuring coding professionals' baseline knowledge will shorten the learning curve, improve coding accuracy and productivity, prepare for educational needs, and accelerate the realization of benefits of the new coding systems. AHIMA plans to provide self-assessment tools and other resources suitable for skill assessment.
   - Review ICD-10-CM coding guidelines, ICD-10-PCS reference manual, and other ICD-10 educational materials to identify areas where increased clinical knowledge will be needed.
   - Use information from coding professional knowledge gap assessment to develop

individualized education plans for improving clinical knowledge to ensure it meets the requirements of ICD-10-CM and ICD-10-PCS.

- If outsourced staff are used for coding, communicate with the companies that provide these services concerning their plans for ICD-10 related training.

- Consider having the coding personnel practice coding a few records using ICD-10-CM and ICD-10-PCS to increase familiarity with the new coding systems.

  - Download ICD-10-CM information at www.cdc.gov/nchs/about/otheract/icd9/icd10cm.htm
  - Download ICD-10-PCS information at http://www.cms.hhs.gov/ICD9 ProviderDiagnosticCodes/08_ICD10.asp

Documentation Improvement

1. Conduct medical record documentation assessments through an internal or external review process.

- Evaluate random samples of various types of medical records to determine adequacy of documentation to support the required level of detail in new coding systems. (AHIMA will be developing a clinical documentation assessment tool to assist with this process.)

- Identify documentation deficiencies and develop a priority list of diagnoses and procedures requiring more granularity or other changes in data capture and recording.

- Identify target segments of medical staff that would benefit from focused education to adapt their documentation practices to what is required for the new systems.

2. Implement a documentation improvement program to address deficiencies identified during the review process and a plan to prevent recurrence.
   - Designate a physician champion to assist in physician education.
   - Identify target segments of medical staff that would benefit from focused education about their documentation practices.
   - Educate medical staff about medical record documentation requirements required by the new coding systems through specific examples, emphasizing the value of more concise data capture for optimal results and better data quality.
   - Monitor documentation for evidence of improvement, identify areas still requiring assistance, and educate medical staff to eliminate remaining deficiencies.

3. Report summary of documentation assessment related to the use of ICD-10 and the achieved progress in improvements to senior management.

Phase 2—Overall Implementation

This stage involves three major tasks: implementation of required IS changes, follow-up assessment of documentation practices, and increasing education of the organization's coding professionals. Also include any items carried over from Phase 1.

Target Audience

- HIM managers
- IS personnel
- Medical staff
- Coding professionals
- Business associates
- Vendors
- Data users

Goals

Organizationwide Implementation Strategy

1. Follow-up with readiness status of payers and other business associates by contacting payers and other business associates for an updated status on their progress toward preparing for ICD-10 implementation.

2. Develop strategies to minimize problems during transition.
   - Assess impact of reduced code assignment productivity on the organization's accounts receivable status.
     - What is the anticipated impact on code assignment through-put?

(Implementation variables that can affect productivity include the amount and level of preparation, extent of coding staff education and credentials, individual code assignment experience and knowledge of anatomy and disease processes, extent of training, quality of medical record documentation, and organizational size and complexity.)

- How long is coding professional productivity expected to be reduced?
- What steps could be taken to reduce the impact of decreased coding professional productivity?
  . Eliminate coding backlogs prior to ICD-10 implementation.
  . Use outsourced personnel for coding to assist with workload during the initial implementation period.
  . Prioritize medical records to be coded.
  . Additional training prior to implementation to improve confidence levels and minimize slow downs.
  . Additional efforts to improve the clarity of medical record documentation.
  . Use of electronic tools to support the code assignment process.
• Assess impact of decreased coding accuracy.
  - What is the anticipated impact on coding accuracy with the new code sets?
  - How long is it expected to take for the coding professionals to achieve the same level of proficiency as with ICD-9-CM?

- What steps could be taken to improve coding accuracy?
  . Additional education
  . Increased monitoring during the initial implementation period. (It is important to consider whether the increased monitoring duties be assumed by staff, or if it will it be necessary to contract with a consultant and how use of existing personnel for more frequent and complex assessment of code assignment impacts the overall workflow.)
- Miscellaneous issues—Identify other potential problems during the transition and implement strategies to reduce potential negative impact.

3. Continue to assess the impact of changing coding systems.
   - Educate data users (e.g., case management, utilization management, quality management, data analysts) on differences in classification of diseases and procedures in the new coding systems, including definitions and code category composition, in order to assess impact on data trends (if not completed in Phase 1).

4. Revise processes, policies, and procedures as appropriate.

5. Provide senior management with regular updates.

6.   Keep affected staff informed through frequent updates regarding progress, next steps, and issue identification and resolution.

7.   Develop a detailed schedule leading up to the point of go-live in order to clearly articulate all key stakeholders' roles and responsibilities.

Information Systems

1.   Follow up with system developers or suppliers regarding their readiness for incorporation of the new code sets.
   • Projected availability of upgrade (still on target with date indicated in Phase 1?)

2.   Determine impact of coding system change on longitudinal data analysis.
   • Where will data mapping occur to link data between the legacy and new coding systems and will outside assistance be needed to create specific mapping applications beyond the maps or crosswalks supplied by the code set developers? Mapping will be needed to cross-reference between pre- and post-crossover periods in order to understand the correlation of ICD-9-CM and ICD-10 data.

3.   Modify the report formats and redesign the forms identified in Phase 1.

4.   Implement and test systems changes, including both in-house and proprietary

systems changes.
- Implement identified in-house systems changes.
- Begin testing both in-house and proprietary systems changes in a coordinated manner.
- Test completed in-house changes.
- Test information systems changes once the system developers have completed the changes.

Education of Coding Professionals

1. HIM coding staff should increase familiarity with the new coding systems and the associated coding guidelines.
- Increase intensity of coder training on the new coding systems and coding guidelines.

Documentation Improvement

1. Continue to assess and improve medical record documentation practices.
- Monitor medical record documentation practices.
- Continue to work with clinicians to improve documentation in areas where deficiencies affect data integrity.

Phase 3—Go-Live Preparation

This stage involves several major tasks: finalization of systems changes, testing of claims transactions with payers, intensive education of the organization's coding professionals, monitoring coding accuracy and reimbursement with prospective payment systems results, including the Diagnosis

Related Group (DRG) assignment. Also include any items carried over from Phase 2.

Target Audience

- HIM managers
- Information systems personnel
- Payers
- Coding professionals
- Vendors
- Financial management (including accounting and billing personnel)

Goals

Organizationwide Implementation Strategy

1. Conduct testing of claims transactions with payers.
   - Six months prior to implementation, test ICD-10 components of claims transactions with payers.

2. Assess potential reimbursement impact of new coding systems.
   - Evaluate potential DRG shifts.
   - Evaluate changes in case mix index.
   - Communicate with payers on anticipated changes in reimbursement schedules or payment policies.

3. Provide senior management with regular updates as to project status.

4. Keep key staff informed through frequent updates regarding progress, next steps, and issue identification and resolution. This could be initially conducted through weekly meetings, e-mail communications, with more frequent communication (perhaps daily) as the go-live date gets closer.

5. Review and modify the detailed schedule leading up to the point of go-live in order to clearly articulate all key stakeholders' roles and responsibilities during the last couple of weeks.

Information Systems

1. Finalize systems changes and complete testing of these changes.
    - Complete all necessary in-house systems changes.
    - Confirm with vendor(s) that changes/ upgrades in vendor systems have been completed.
    - Finish testing the changes.
    - Make modifications in response to the results of the testing and conduct regression testing.

Education of Coding Professionals

1. Complete intensive coding professional education and education of other users previously identified as requiring education.
    - Three to six months prior to implementation, all coding staff should complete intensive education on applying the new coding

systems (the estimated amount of training is 24–40 hours, depending on whether coding professionals require both ICD-10-CM and ICD-10-PCS education).

- Document completion of this training in personnel files.
- To ensure the quality and consistency of ICD-10 education, it is recommended that training be conducted by an AHIMA-certified trainer.
- Sources of training include:
    - Distance education courses
    - Audio seminars or Web-based in-services
    - Self-directed learning using printed materials or electronic tools
    - Traditional classroom training by a certified trainer
- Communicate with companies supplying contracted coding staff to ensure they have received the necessary education and ask for documentation to confirm that training has occurred and has been provided by a qualified source (e.g., AHIMA-certified trainer).
- Implement the identified education plan for users of coded data and document completion of the training in their personnel files.

GO LIVE!

Phase 4—Post-implementation

This phase consists of monitoring coding accuracy for reimbursement, other data management impact, coding productivity, and continuing with appropriate coding professional training.

Target Audience

- HIM managers
- Information systems personnel
- Payers
- Coding professionals
- Medical staff
- Senior management
- Others, depending on identified problems to be resolved
- Financial management (including accounting, and billing personnel)

Goals

Organizationwide Implementation Strategy

1. The ICD-10 steering committee should continue to meet regularly to share information regarding implementation progress, including monitoring of the status of issue resolution, discussing lessons learned, and identifying best practices. These meetings should continue until the committee feels they are no longer necessary.

2. Keep key staff informed regarding issue identification and resolution through weekly updates or institution of a Web-based issue

tracking system that would allow staff to check the status of an issue at any time.

3. Train or re-train staff; continue budgetary planning for training of staff.
   - Train new staff.
   - Train staff unavailable during previous training.
   - Provide re-training or additional training as needed.

4. Assess the reimbursement impact of the new system, provide education to staff on reimbursement issues, and monitor case mix and reimbursement group (e.g., DRGs) assignment.
   - Work closely with payers to resolve payment issues, such as claims denials or rejections.
   - Communicate with payers on anticipated changes in reimbursement schedules or payment policies.
   - Analyze changes in case mix index.
   - Concurrently review case mix or reimbursement groups (e.g., DRGs, HHRGs) and diagnosis and procedure code assignments.
   - Analyze shifts in reimbursement groups.
   - Provide education and feedback regarding reimbursement issues to staff.

5. Resolve post-implementation problems as expeditiously as possible.
   - The interdisciplinary steering committee should follow up on post-implementation problems, such as claims denials or rejections or coding backlogs.

- Work with internal staff or external entities as appropriate to resolve problems as expeditiously as possible.

6. Monitor coding professional productivity.
   - Develop plans to address coding professional backlogs such as contracting to outsource coding professionals.

7. Maintain communication with payers and resolve any problems.

8. Keep senior management informed of identified issues and progress in resolving them through pre-scheduled standing meetings or weekly updates.

Information Systems

1. Monitor and respond to any information systems problems or issues.

Education of Coding Professionals

1. Post-implementation, monitor coding accuracy closely and initiate corrective action as necessary, such as providing additional education.

Documentation Improvement

1. Continue to monitor medical record documentation and work with medical staff on documentation improvement strategies if needed.

Acknowledgements

June Bronnert, RHIA, CCS, CCS-P
Donald T. Mon, PhD
Rita Scichilone, MHSA, RHIA, CCS, CCS-P
Allison Viola, MBA, RHIA

Reference

AHIMA's Coding Products and Services Team. "Destination 10: Healthcare Organization Preparation for ICD-10-CM and ICD-10-PCS." (AHIMA Practice Brief). *Journal of AHIMA* 75, no.3 (March 2004): 56A-D.

References

AHIMA e-HIM Workgroup on the Transition to ICD-10-CM/PCS. 2009. Planning organizational transition to ICD-10-CM/PCS. *Journal of AHIMA* 80(10):72-77. http://library.ahima.org/xpedio/groups/public/documents/ahima/bok1_044964.hcsp?dDocName=bok1_044964.

AHIMA e-HIM Workgroup on the Transition to ICD-10-CM/PCS. 2009. Transitioning ICD-10-CM/PCS Data Management Processes. *Journal of AHIMA* 80(10):66-70. http://library.ahima.org/xpedio/groups/public/documents/ahima/bok1_044963.hcsp?dDocName=bok1_044963.

American Hospital Association and American Health Information Management Association. 2003. ICD-10-CM Field Testing Project: Report on Findings. http://www.ahima.org/icd10/documents/FinalStudy.pdf.

Bowman, S., Zeisset, A., and L. Czarkowski. 2008. Webinar: Beginning the Transition to ICD-10. Chicago: AHIMA. [Available to members only.]

Barta, A., et al. 2008. ICD-10-CM Primer. *Journal of AHIMA* 79(5):64-66. http://www.ahima.org/infocenter/documents/ICD-10resourceslinks.pdf.

Bowman, S. 2007. Brushing Up On ICD-10-PCS. *Journal of AHIMA* 78(9):108-112. http://www.ahima.org/infocenter/documents/ICD-10resourceslinks.pdf.

Bowman, S., and A. Zeisset. ICD-10 Preparation Checklist. Updated June 2007. AHIMA. http://www.ahima.org/icd10/ICD-10PreparationChecklist.mht.

Butler, R. 2008. Crossing the Bridge to ICD-10: Using the General Equivalence Mappings (GEMs) to Create an ICD-10 Ready Workplace. 2008 AHIMA Convention Proceedings. http://www.ahima.org/infocenter/documents/ICD-10resourceslinks.pdf.

Butler, R., and R. Mills. 2009. ICD-10 Reimbursement Mappings: New Mappings from CMS Help Organizations in the Transition to ICD-10. *Journal of AHIMA* 80(4):66-69.

Butler, R., and P. Wilson. 2006. Navigating Uncharted Territory: Mapping ICD-9-CM to ICD-10-CM and ICD-10-PCS. AHIMA's 78th National Convention and Exhibit Proceedings. http://www.ahima.org/infocenter/documents/ICD-10resourceslinks.pdf.

Butler, R. The ICD-10 General Equivalence Mappings: Bridging the Translation Gap from ICD-9. *Journal of AHIMA* 78(9):84-86. http://www.ahima.org/infocenter/documents/ICD-10resourceslinks.pdf.

Butler, R. 2008. Where the Rubber Meets the Road: Application of ICD-10-PCS Coding in Complex Surgical Scenarios. 2008 AHIMA Convention Proceedings.

Campbell, J.R., and M. Imel. 2005. The Function of Rule-Based Mapping within Integrated Terminology Management. AHIMA's 77th National Convention and Exhibit Proceedings.

Centers for Medicare & Medicaid Services.
2009. ICD-10 Procedure Coding System
(ICD-10-PCS). http://www.cms.hhs.gov/
ICD10.
Code Tables and Index
ICD-10-PCS Reference Manual
ICD-10-PCS Slides
Development of the ICD-10 Procedure Coding
System

Centers for Medicare & Medicaid Services. 2009.
General Equivalence Mappings: ICD-9-CM To
and From ICD-10-CM and ICD-10-PCS Fact
Sheet. http://www.cms.hhs.gov/MLNProducts/
downloads/ICD-10_GEM_factsheet.pdf.

Centers for Medicare & Medicaid Services.
2009. Second in Series: General Equivalence
Mappings: ICD-9-CM To and From
ICD-10-CM and ICD-10-PCS Fact Sheet.
http://www.cms.hhs.gov/ICD10/Downloads/
secondinGEMseries.pdf.

Centers for Medicare & Medicaid Services. 2009.
Procedure Code Set General Equivalence
Mappings, ICD-10-PCS to ICD-9-CM and
ICD-9-CM to ICD-10-PCS, 2009 Version
Documentation and User's Guide. http://www.
cms.hhs.gov/ICD10/01m_2009_ICD10PCS.asp.

Centers for Medicare & Medicaid Services. 2008.
Medicare Learning Network (MLN) Number
SE0832: The ICD-10 Clinical Modification/
Procedure Coding System (CM/PCS)—The
Next Generation of Coding. http://www.cms.
hhs.gov/MLNMattersArticles/downloads/
SE0832.pdf.

Centers for Medicare & Medicaid Services. 2009. Medicare Learning Network (MLN) Number 902143: ICD-10-CM/PCS Myths & Facts. http://www.cms.hhs.gov/MLNProducts/downloads/ICD-10-CM_PCS_Myths&Facts.pdf.

Centers for Medicare & Medicaid Services. 2009. Sponsored call: Introduction to ICD-10-CM/PCS for Physician Specialty Group Representatives. http://www.cms.hhs.gov/ICD10/Downloads/ICD-10-CM_PCS_for_Physician_Spec_Group_Rep_Presentation.pdf.

Centers for Medicare & Medicaid Services. 2008. Sponsored call: ICD-10 Overview Presentation. http://www.cms.hhs.gov/ContractorLearningResources/Downloads/ICD-10_Overview_Presentation.pdf.

Department of Health and Human Services. 2004. The Costs and Benefits of Moving to the ICD-10 Code Sets. Santa Monica, CA: RAND Corporation. http://www.rand.org/pubs/technical_reports/2004/RAND_TR132.pdf.

Department of Health and Human Services. 2009. HIPAA Administrative Simplifications: Modifications to Medical Data Code Set Standards to Adopt ICD-10-PCS and ICD-10-PCS: Final Rule. 45 CFR Part 162. *Federal Register* 74(11):3328–62. http://edocket.access.gpo.gov/2009/pdf/E9-743.pdf.

Zeisset, A. 2010. Edited by International Classification of Diseases (ICD) and the U.S. Modifications. Chapter 2 in *Healthcare Code Sets, Clinical Terminologies, and Classification Systems*, 2nd ed. Edited by K. Giannangelo. Chicago: AHIMA.

Hazelwood, A, and C. Venable. 2009. *ICD-10-CM and ICD-10-PCS Preview*, 2nd ed. Chicago: AHIMA.

Lau, L. M., and J.R. Campbell. 2003. Putting Standards to Work: Vocabulary Implementation in the Real World. AMIA 2003 Annual Symposium.

McBride, S., et al. 2006. Data Mapping. *Journal of AHIMA* 77(2):44-48. [Expanded online edition available to members only.]

National Center for Health Statistics. 2009. *2009 Release, International Classification of Diseases, Tenth Revision, Clinical Modification (ICD-10-CM)*. http://www.cdc.gov/nchs/icd/icd10cm.htm.

National Center for Health Statistics. 2009. *General Equivalence Mapping Files (ICD-10-CM)*. http://www.cdc.gov/nchs/icd/icd10cm.htm#09update.

Resources

Governmental Resources

Centers for Medicare & Medicaid Services. 2009 and 2008 ICD-10 CMS Sponsored Calls (discussion materials and transcripts). http://www.cms.hhs.gov/ICD10/06a_2009_CMS_Sponsored_Calls.asp. http://www.cms.hhs.gov/ICD10/07_Sponsored_Calls.asp.

Centers for Medicare & Medicaid Services. ICD-10 General Information. http://www.cms.hhs.gov/ICD10.

Centers for Medicare & Medicaid Services. ICD-10 Educational Resources (fact sheets). http://www.cms.hhs.gov/ICD10/05_Educational_Resources.asp.

Department of Health and Human Services. 2008. HIPAA Administrative Simplifications: Modifications to Medical Data Code Set Standards to Adopt ICD-10-PCS and ICD-10-PCS: Proposed Rule. 45 CFR Parts 160 and 162. *Federal Register* 73(164): 49796–832. http://edocket.access.gpo.gov/2008/pdf/E8-19298.pdf.

National Center for Health Statistics. General ICD-10 Information. http://www.cdc.gov/.

Code Sets: ICD-10-CM

2009 ICD-10-CM. http://www.cdc.gov/.
- ICD-10-CM Index to Diseases and Injuries
- ICD-10-CM Tabular List of Diseases and Injuries
  - Instructional Notations
- Official Guidelines for Coding and Reporting
  (Draft 2009)
- Mapping ICD-9-CM to ICD-10-CM and
  ICD-10-CM to ICD-9-CM
- Documentation and Users Guide
- Code Descriptions
- Changes to ICD-10-CM Descriptions File

Code Sets: ICD-10-PCS

The index and tabular sections of ICD-10-PCS can be obtained at http://www.cms.hhs.gov/ICD10/. This site also provides the ICD-10-PCS Reference Manual, forward and backwards mappings between ICD-9-CM and ICD-10-PCS, and draft coding guidelines (located in the Reference Manual.) Also available is a very helpful PowerPoint presentation explaining the coding system, and a document called: Development of the ICD-10 Procedure Coding System (ICD-10-PCS.) Much of the detailed information provided earlier in this chapter is derived from the Development of the ICD-10 Procedure Coding System document available on the Internet.

In addition to the online manual, ICD-10-PCS provides an ICD-10-PCS Reference Manual (including the coding guidelines). These files are all available at the CMS Web site referenced above. A significant improvement was made in 2009 by adding Body Part Keys in the reference section of the online ICD-10-PCS to assist with anatomical terms in ICD-10-PCS. The components of these various resources are listed below.

- 2009 Code Tables and Index
  - ICD-10-PCS 2009 Tables
  - References
    . List of Sections
    . Global Root Operations (Sections 0–9)
    . Global Root Types (Sections B–H)
    . Body Part Key by PCS Description
    . Body Part Key by Anatomical Term
    . Medical and Surgical Approaches
    . Type Qualifier (Character 5)/Includes for Physical Rehabilitation and Diagnostic Audiology (F)
    . Mental Health (G)—Type— Explanation
    . Substance Abuse Treatment—Type— Explanation
  - Index
- 2009 ICD-10-PCS Reference Manual
  - Chapter 1: ICD-10-PCS Overview
  - Chapter 2: Procedures in the Medical and Surgical Section
  - Chapter 3: Procedures in the Medical and Surgical-related Sections
  - Chapter 4: Procedures in the Ancillary Sections
  - Appendix A: ICD-10-PCS Definitions
    . Root Operations
    . Approaches
  - Appendix B: ICD-10-PCS Draft Coding Guidelines

. General
. Medical and Surgical Section (Section 0)
. Other Medical and Surgical-related
Sections (Sections 1–9)
- 2009 ICD-10-PCS Slides
  - PCS2009 Slides—PowerPoint presentation
- 2009 Development of the ICD-10 Procedure
  Coding System
- 2009 Version—What's New
- 2009 Mapping ICD-10-PCS to ICD-9-CM
  and ICD-9-CM to ICD-10-PCS; User Guide,
  Reimbursement Guide, Diagnosis and
  Procedures
- 2009 Code Descriptions
- 2009 Addendum

AHIMA Resources

In addition to the AHIMA items referenced
throughout this book (and listed above), AHIMA
has many resources on its ICD-10 Web site. Much
of the information is available to all, while select
resources are available to AHIMA members
through the AHIMA's Body of Knowledge. http://
www.ahima.org/icd10.

About ICD-10. http://www.ahima.org/icd10/
about.html.
AHIMA Leads the Way. http://www.ahima.org/
icd10/ahima-icd10.html.
AHIMA's Advocacy Efforts. http://www.ahima.
org/icd10/advocacy-efforts.html.
Benefits Outweigh the Costs. http://www.ahima.
org/icd10/benefits-vs-costs.html.

Collection of articles in the Body of Knowledge on ICD-10. http://www.ahima.org/icd10/links.html.

Educational Opportunities for ICD-10. http://www.ahima.org/icd10/education-training.html.

Frequently Asked Questions. http://www.ahima.org/icd10/icd-10-faqs.html.

ICD-10-CM/PCS Final Rule. http://www.ahima.org/icd10/icd-10-final-rule.html.

ICD-TEN e-newsletter. http://www.ahima.org/images/newsletters/ICDTen/subscribe.html.

Links & Other Resources. http://www.ahima.org/icd10/links.html.

Networking Opportunities and Speaker Requests. http://www.ahima.org/icd10/icd-10-talk.html.

Preparing for ICD-10. http://www.ahima.org/icd10/preparing-for-icd-10.html.

Press Release & News. http://www.ahima.org/icd10/press-releases-news.html.

Purposes of Classifications and Terminologies. http://www.ahima.org/icd10/classifications-terminologies.html.

Understanding ICD-10. http://www.ahima.org/icd10/understanding-icd-10.html.

The Value of ICD-10. http://www.ahima.org/icd10/value-icd-10.html.

What is ICD-10? http://www.ahima.org/icd10/what-is-icd-10.html.

Why is ICD-9 being replaced? http://www.ahima.org/icd10/why-replace-icd-9.html.

Notes